I0425999

# THE MENOPAUSE SUCCESS TRIANGLE

*A Practical Guide to Living a Healthy, Happy Menopause Life*

## BY

## Kris T. Smith

ISBN-13: 978-1492269021
ISBN-10: 1492269026

# TABLE OF CONTENTS

# -SIX- EATING PALEO for Menopause Health &

# Wellness _____ 192

# FOREWORD

## Carrie T. Pierce, Menopauserus.com

Never before has there been a man on this planet who understands the midlife female body—and the menopause process—like Kris T. Smith!

Kris is blessed with amazing insight, profound knowledge, wisdom, and laser-like clarity. When it comes to helping women struggling through the menopause process, his new book, "The Menopause Success Triangle," simply ROCKS!

We all know what an amazing time of profound transformation that menopause can be. Yet, all too often, the blessings are overlooked because they lie buried in a tangled mass of physical and emotional symptoms, fatigue, loss of self-esteem, and a sense of grief and despair...

Kris innately understands this conundrum, and stands ready to throw lifeline after lifeline, leading the menopausal reader to a place that ultimately reveals her best self: her best health, her best body, her best vitality, and her best beauty.

If you're in your midlife years, this book is a MUST READ! Place yourself in Kris' care, and find yourself amazingly transformed in just a few short weeks!

> - Carrie E. Pierce, Founder and President
> *Menopauserus.com*
> Host, "Magnificent Menopause and Beyond©"

# FOREWORD

## Dr. Eve Agee

If you are ready to have more energy and feel better during menopause and beyond, then read and use the strategies in this wonderful book by my friend Kris T. Smith. Kris is an excellent guide to helping women become fit and healthy during their 40s, 50s and 60s.

You're going to love what you find in these pages.

-   Dr. Eve Agee, Best Selling Author
    *The Uterine Health Companion: A Holistic Guide to Lifelong Wellness*)

## FOREWORD
### Greg Kalafatic–Nutrition Expert

It started out as a fantasy.

Have you ever gone back to your elementary school yearbook and realized that you had the most vivid imagination when you read the answer to:

*What do you want to be when you grow up?*

Back then, without hesitation, I wrote: a professional football player. It turns out that, although I didn't know it back then, that answer actually stood for something more powerful to me, like an unlinked analogy.

Deep down I knew that there was something special, deep within me. It was my willingness to work hard in life, whether on academics, physical activity, or just making people laugh.

I had such a strong desire to succeed that I progressed in most facets of my life every year (except for shyness with the ladies). I grew up in a great home with parents who possessed amazing love for their children and gave unto us (my siblings as well) whatever they could. Friends and family praised and recognized me as a special man, someone who was kind, gentle, compassionate, and ambitious, destined to shock the world. I always seemed to make it in the cards each year.

You would think life would have been a breeze for me, having so much support, but somewhere I lost my way, my drive, my spirit ... MYSELF!

I lost my mother to lung cancer, my father to depression, my siblings and relatives to disconnections. Life crashed down around me. I had no direction, no way out ... a numb life. I didn't turn to drugs or alcohol. It was worse than that. I succumbed to Giving Up and losing all hope.

Then, I met Kris. I started my career in personal training and nutrition, and my life began to turn around. Kris saw that spark in me and knew that, with a little guidance and mentoring, I had something special to offer. He pushed me, drove me, inspired me, empowered me, and at times even ticked me off.

But his belief in me allowed me to turn to that very passion and dream that I had had back in elementary school. Not to be a professional football player, exactly, but to be someone whom people watched, looked up to, followed, and were inspired by as they made important changes in their lives.

Nicknamed "Mr. Nutrition" by a community of men and women who just needed compassion and guidance, I have found my way again. More than ever, I am excited to be that young man who dreamed of greatness and of making an impact on the world.

Now it's your turn to be filled with hope and inspiration from Kris. You may be facing a similar, unknown path as you begin menopause. You may be dreading the fact that "life is over," or thinking that "life will never be the same."

Kris is that special person who will shock any woman facing or about to face menopause. At first, these thoughts may go through your mind:

What does a 35-year-old African-American male who walks with a disability know about menopause? He has never experienced pain like "we" have, right? He can't possibly understand what we are feeling, right?

On the contrary, when you hear Kris' story, and feel his compassion for creating permanent change for women who are battling with their bodies, you'll erase those doubts and become a disciple of his work.

You won't need to follow him blindly. He invites you to walk side by side with him as he supports you, and witnesses the transformations in your life. You will come to believe, to live, and to love again.

Kris has cracked the Menopause Success Triangle by being vulnerable. In this book and in his daily work, he opens up his life to you, learns exactly what it is you are facing, and then offers a solution. He is a true, indefatigable survivor.

Over the last 6 years, I have watched Kris grow and transform into the man he is today. I saw Kris wake up from a dream with those three fateful words on his mind: *My Menopause Fix!* I saw him seek out the top experts in the field of women's menopausal health, read countless books and medical journals, write hundreds of blog posts and articles, put together a life-changing event called the World Menopause Summit, and now write this very book that is filled with so much hope, it can't help but change your life.

I am happy to call Kris a best friend, a brother, and a mentor.

If you pick up this book, it's because you too had a dream, and are seeking to put your life back together. You've found a great partner with whom to face the sometimes overwhelming territory of menopause.

Kris is the Menopause Savior that this world has been waiting for. Open your mind to the possibilities that Kris offers, and you, too, will find yourself again.

With Love,

> Greg Kalafatic
> "Mr. Nutrition"

# FOREWORD
## AnnaMaria DeMaria

My journey began 5 years ago. I was 44 years old, a Registered Medical Assistant (RMA) in adult cardiology, and suddenly in need of taking control of my life and body as I entered peri-menopause. I found a man (yes, man!) who changed my life: Kris T. Smith. I knew within 5 minutes of meeting him that he "saw the female body like no other male."

I was suffering from terrible hot flashes, insomnia, and fatigue. My diet was poor, and I no longer felt comfortable in my own skin. But how could he possibly help?

Kris had an innovative program that helped me to regain control through exercise and proper nutrition. But I realized that he couldn't help me all alone. I had to choose to commit to it, as well, in order to be successful. I needed to change my mindset, and make the changes.

So, without skepticism, I welcomed him as my trainer, my mentor, and my friend. Kris was a constant support for me, inspiring me to health. He encouraged me to believe in myself, and assisted me to see life differently. I spent three days with him in the gym every week, worked hard, and diligently changed my eating habits. I consider myself one of his many success stories after immersing myself in his innovative program. I know that, no matter what your age, it is possible to live a happy, healthier life.

- AnnaMaria DeMaria,
"The MenoDiva"
RMA, CPT, editor/blogger

# PREFACE

I've had to overcome a lot of obstacles in my own life. I was born with my right leg four inches shorter than my left. I didn't have either a hamstring or quadriceps on that leg, so the doctors told me that I'd spend my life in a wheelchair, never able to participate in sports like a normal child. I did not accept this diagnosis. Even as a kid I knew that, to have a normal, happy life, I'd need a rock-solid mindset. I had to teach myself that I could achieve anything that my mind could conceive or believe.

I found a way to be really successful and to work in a profession that I love, based around fitness, health, and strength training, with incredible clients that I can help every day. But the journey to creating that life was pretty daunting. I had to figure out how to meet obstacles like my leg and not just overcome them, but turn them into amazing new opportunities. There were plenty of times growing up when I was embarrassed about how I looked, self-conscious about how I moved, and temporarily psyched out about what I could or couldn't do. I often felt that no one else could possibly understand what I was going through, and that nobody would get how it felt to be me.

Those experiences, including the negative ones, really made me an ideal coach and trainer for women who are dealing with the discomforts and challenges of menopause. I've been training and coaching women in my private fitness practice for six years now.

***In fact, 90-95% of my clients are women, and in the course of our sessions together, they began to share with me their physical and emotional struggles with the peri-menopause life stage***.

I researched and developed a lot of my ideas for this book and the MyMenopauseFix blog through listening to my clients, aged 42-60.

I have accumulated a wealth of recommendations that have already proven successful in overcoming women's symptoms, and that have significantly reversed their weight gain, lowered their stress levels, and returned them to a positive, forward-looking mindset about this exciting new chapter in their lives.

When I was growing up, and when I encountered physical challenges to my own happiness and well-being, I learned quickly that the key to success began with my mental game. As I began to work with the women that I describe in this book, I related immediately to their feelings of confusion, doubt, lack of motivation, worry, and defeat. I found that I was a perfect person to coach them through their struggles. I always began by addressing the ways that they *thought*, and by coaching around what they *believed* they could do or want.

*For me, success has always come down to the 6 inches between my ears.*

*My clients have shown me that your MIND will dictate your success in life, along with how you create your own transformative, healthy experience of menopause*.

I have been fortunate to have clients who have been very vocal about the things that have helped them through their menopause process. In looking at my client logs from the past seven years, I saw clearly what worked to help women to lower their stress levels, to gain confidence, lose weight, reduce pain, and increase libido. The women that I work with have regular victories because of the lifestyle changes that they have adopted during menopause.

I decided that I wanted more women to learn how to create a lifestyle that handles peri-menopause and menopause naturally, without Hormone Replacement Therapy, without drugs, and without the many negative side effects that can come with this life transition.

*In this book I give you a plan for success based on my analysis of 780 clients and our work together during 1,700 hours of one-on-one coaching.*

I share how women can lessen the severity of all 34 menopause symptoms by building an active lifestyle, eating cleanly, and reducing stress through the process of lowering their body's cortisol levels, that also bring on belly fat in middle age. Gaining weight is not inevitable, just because you turn 45!

I wrote this book for the same reason that I work with my clients on Long Island: *__I love people.__* I love helping women, and I love to see the success and change that comes to those who learn the lessons I teach. It is so inspiring to see each and every one of them incorporate these ideas and directions into this *new chapter of their life* called MENOPAUSE.

# INTRODUCTION
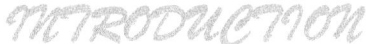

I want you to approach this book the same way that I approach life.

***It all starts with your mindset.***

The more positive, open, and optimistic that you are about the new experiences that accompany menopause, the more you will succeed in co-creating a fresh "life chapter" that is exciting, stress-free, and fantastic.

This book is addressed to any woman in the process of peri-menopause or post-menopause who wants to tackle the **weight gain, stress**, and necessary **changes in nutrition and exercise** that accompany those ten+ years when menopause takes over a woman's body.

***It addresses fitness and lifestyle management for every woman's menopausal health.***

Have you already noticed that what you did, how you ate, and where you were in your 20s and 30s no longer works for you? My mission is to support you—in your new place—with this book.

I believe that we can always improve our mindset: through affirmations, which I discuss in chapter 4; and through staying positive, reading positive books, listening to tapes, being around positive people, and firing the negative people out of our lives.

My own life has been a series of obstacles that I've needed to overcome. Success has always begun first **with my mind,** before I dealt with any of the physical or practical problems that arose.

So I believe that, *as you embrace these ideas that I prescribe for a more positive mindset*, you'll be able to move forward smoothly through peri-menopause and menopause.

> ▶ **You'll regain your composure**
> ▶ **Regain your confidence**
> ▶ **Regain your strength ... AND**

▶ You'll love yourself inside and out

▶ Become more physically active

▶ Feel more mentally alert, and

▶ Learn *what* to eat *when* and *how much*, in order to fuel your body

**You'll discover that you can live the life that you want to live.**

I'll illustrate what I know can work for you, too, through the stories of some of the great women that I've coached. Each one of my sample clients had very specific symptoms and experiences as they went through menopause. And each one probably has things in common with you.

- You'll hear about one client who found that my recommendations about changing her nutrition helped her to get over the hump of her symptoms.
- Another woman loved the way that I put together exercises tailored specifically to her needs, at this unique point in her life.
- *Each* woman appreciated the way that I bring a positive mindset to our workouts. Positivity

inspires them in the same way that it has inspired me.

*Daily, I see how each woman's positive attitude has helped her to reduce stress in very direct, strategic ways*.

This book begins by laying out for you some foundations about menopause facts, myths, and key symptoms. It also shares my strong beliefs about how to build an open, supportive menopause mindset for yourself, one that will help you to stay positive, to embrace your inner beauty, and to prepare you to take on all of the recommendations and actions that I describe.

In the rest of the book, you will find strategies for changing your approach to diet, exercise, and stress.

*I'm going to share my Menopause Success Triangle. My Secret Sauce. Chapter 5 is the ANSWER to ALL OF YOUR MENOPAUSE PRAYERS! It's all about how to tackle, survive, and truly ENJOY this time in your life.*

Along the way, I will introduce you to some of the great women that I've worked with. Their specific stories and examples are going to inspire you to get the most out of this book. Through them, I'll explain all of my positive ideas, and describe the advice and strategies that I have to offer. I've chosen to tell you about these clients because I think that their true stories really illustrate best how my principles can work for you.

I invite you to focus in on whatever elements of my program will assist you best at your own personal stage in life. I know that all of the information here is awesome, and that everything I share has proven to be successful with hundreds of clients over thousands of hours of coaching and training. But it may not all apply to you: ***please target the parts of your life that could benefit from whatever I have to offer.***

I will keep coming back to my belief that CHANGING YOUR LIFESTYLE is more important to a successful menopause than any medication or synthetic drug.

In fact, here's another mindset that I really hope you'll change, as you work through this book:

**Drugs aren't the only legitimate way to treat this** or any other change in your body's physical and emotional state.

In the United States, we spend $300 billion each year on drugs: <u>three times what the rest of the world spends</u>, **<u>combined.</u>** We are also the only country other than New Zealand that advertises prescription drugs on TV, and invites you to "ask your doctor" about them.

There isn't anything here that you can't or shouldn't discuss with your doctor.

But for the most part, this is a **natural, pro-active approach to what is a normal, exciting life stage**.

My book and program support the good that you can do for yourself, and assert that your body can and wants to be healthy. Let's help it out—so you feel fantastic!

-ONE-

## 7 Most Common Menopause Symptoms

Menopause is a natural occurrence that visits each woman differently. Similar to the first signs of a young girl's menstrual period and the inception of puberty, **menopause is a life milestone**. It indicates the end of menstruation. Signs of this rite of passage can occur in women as young as 35-40 years old; peri-menopause or the "menopause transition" can commence as early as a woman's late 30s or as late as her early 50s, and last up to a year after her final period.

Peri-menopause lasts up until menopause, which is technically the point at which a woman's ovaries stop releasing eggs. In the last one to two years of peri-menopause, there is acceleration in the physiological decline of estrogen. That decrease in the key reproductive hormone, and other hormones related to it, produces many of the 34 symptoms that women feel and hear so much about.

Hormones Change; Symptoms Appear

The **7 Most Common Menopause Symptoms** that my clients complain to me about are a direct result of changes in their levels of **estrogen** and **progesterone.** These two reproductive hormones are generated by the body in great abundance during a young woman's adolescent years. When pregnancy and reproduction aren't absolutely necessary anymore, the body turns down the level of these key hormones.

These 7 Most Common Symptoms develop in women during peri-menopause, **BUT** *every woman experiences this shift or transition in her own way*.

Let me describe the key challenging symptoms, from my clients' perspective. *See if any of these changes sound familiar...*

**Everything that I talk about below is triggered by hormones**. The physical symptoms. *And* the psychological changes, too. Some hormones are *waning* at this stage of your life. But others *increase* in ways that may cause discomfort, weight gain, and other challenges.

This is the peri-menopause phenomenon. Then: the menopause occurs. Some doctors peg it to a cessation of a woman's period for six or twelve months.

***A woman is in her postmenopausal phase for the rest of her life.***

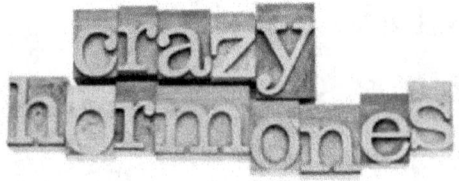

And it's not JUST hormones...!

The severity of this life change for you—*your unique experience of these symptoms—*ALSO depends on various **genetic** and **internal** factors. **Lifestyle and nutrition choices** influence its intensity, too.

Unfortunately, I can't change a woman's genes!

But **I CAN offer specific recommendations and adjustments to your diet and exercise**, ones that really, specifically impact the intensity of these 7 Common Symptoms, along with everything else experienced during menopause.

My clients like Lizz and Deborah joined the majority of my clients in describing the following as the *7 Magic Symptoms* of menopause. They discovered that we could tackle them through natural solutions that lessened their severity. I'll share those with you in my next few chapters.

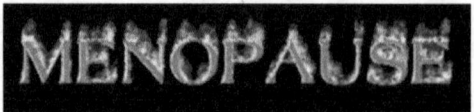

## 1. Hot Flashes—All Day Long, Anytime

This symptom is super common. It is a phenomenon that Lizz described to me as hard to explain *only until you have had your first one*!

For her, it was an intense heat that came on rapidly, often starting in her chest then rising to her neck and face. She would feel beads of perspiration on her forehead, and then sometimes even have rivulets run down her temples for three, four, five minutes, many times each day or week.

Deborah experienced less intense flushes. They did appear in a rush, like Lizz's, but then pulsed and lingered for nearly thirty minutes. Neither woman ever found that their sudden overheating was connected to the weather: it certainly didn't have to be hot outside for them to be suddenly bathing in sweat!

These flashes or flushes or full on heat attacks are scientifically linked to a jolt in your *estrogen* level, which may be connected to the parts of our brain that control internal temperature. The rush of perspiration is our body's attempt to cool you off and bring you back to a neutral, comfortable temperature.

Since the drop and surge of estrogen is the hormonal process at the root of peri-menopause, most every woman has this symptom to some degree. Other doctors add that hot flashes may also be impacted by our levels of **leptin**, a hormone that's produced in the fat cells; hot flashes are additionally exacerbated by changes to blood sugar levels that are shifted by others of your hormones.

For some women, hot flashes come and go.

Other women awaken at night drenched in perspiration, and need to change their clothes.

Maybe you, too, have found yourself with wet-looking pants in painfully public places.

Thankfully, these flashes do abate as your estrogen eventually tapers off. They disappear once your periods stop completely.

In the meantime, however, Lizz, Deborah, and many others needed to make some lifestyle changes in order to handle their excessive perspiring. I'll get to those soon … **Read on!**

## 2. Weight Gain

Lizzette had **gone up four dress sizes** during menopause in her mid-40s before she came to work with me as her coach. Jillian **suddenly gained 15 pounds**. And in the two years after her menopause, Barbara B. **gained 25-30 pounds**.

There is no question here: a woman over 45 <u>will</u> experience that **her metabolism slows down with age**.

It's a fact.

Dr. Madelyn Fernstrom of the Weight Management Center at the University of Pittsburgh Medical Center says, "Compared to age 25, you'll burn

200 fewer calories at 45. Do nothing, and you could gain *eight to twelve pounds a year."*

Your metabolism is slated to decrease at a rate of approximately 5% each decade.

Lizzette said to me that she had been eating the same amount, or less, as she always had throughout her 30s, but was gaining weight anyway.

Barbara looked around at other women aged 50-59 and found that about 30% of them weren't just overweight: they were obese.

Like nearly 90% of all women in menopause, Lizzette and Barbara had *gained weight from a shift in their hormones* *coupled with* *other metabolic changes* that come with age. In addition, Lizzette found that she tended to *retain water weight* during peri-menopause, because of her hormonal fluctuations.

Here are **3 TOP REASONS** why these women and others of my clients *gained weight* during this time of their life. Do any of these things apply to you?

**A. You are less likely to exercise.** 60% of adults are not active enough, and this tendency increases with age.

**B. You lose muscle mass,** which decreases your resting metabolism, making it easier to gain weight.

**C. Your aerobic capacity declines,** which is the rate at which you can use energy during exercise. In order to use the same energy as in the past and achieve weight loss, you will need to increase the amount of time and intensity at which you exercise, no matter what your past activity levels.

One thing to know is that, like Barbara's, *some of your weight gain in peri-menopause is just*

***appearance-based:*** it is related to water retention and the bloating that comes from decreased progesterone levels. While this isn't fat-related, many women still feel uncomfortable about how it may change the ways that their clothes fit.

In medical terms, water retention is known as ***edema,*** and it occurs when water leaks into body tissues from the blood. Under normal circumstances, fluid drains out of these tissues through the lymphatic system, which is the body's network of tubes that removes waste and extraneous material; the fluid is then emptied back into the bloodstream.

Menopause is one of the reasons why women experience water retention, but there are also a number of other reasons. The fact that the body is holding on to water can signal the fact that it thinks that it is not getting enough water in order to function properly.

Some believe that, since your body isn't releasing enough water, the first thing to do is to increase the amount of water that you drink daily. Most people are going to tell you to reduce the amount of salt that you are taking in, too, and this may help to a certain extent.

But **what I explained to Barbara is that too much salt without enough water is going to cause problems** with water retention. And **too much water without enough salt is going to cause _another_ problem**, a reduction in the vitamins and minerals that are contained inside of your body.

*Menopauseatoz.com* explains that water retention during menopause is generally not due to some serious underlying condition, but simply because **the kidneys get tired of working so hard** and, hence, fluid is retained.

Contrary to popular medical advice that you should drink lots of fluids, I sometimes suggest that women like Barbara **cut back on their fluid intake**, just to see if that helps to eliminate some of their water-weight gain.

*If you notice that your hands, fingers, feet, and ankles are swelling consistently, however, something other than simple water-weight gain may be going on. If you press down on your skin and it remains dented afterwards, this may indicate edema, and you should check with your physician.*

With Lizzette and Jillian, I helped them to get rid of water retention and kick up their health level by coaching them how to ***fully hydrate their body.*** I have my clients drink half of their body weight every day in ounces of water. (So—when a client weighs 150 pounds, I have her drink 75 ounces daily, or two full liter bottles, plus a cup of mint tea.) I also have them take a pinch of natural sea salt every time that they drink a glass of water. Try it! If you do this every day, you should begin to notice a difference in the amount of water that you retain.

I have a series of meal and exercise plans in later chapters that are specifically designed to help you to lose this menopause weight; they will help to increase your metabolism, too.

**You'll be able to join Lizzette, Barbara and so many others in keeping your weight down during and after your menopause.**

### 3. Insomnia and Poor Quality of Sleep

During menopause, a woman's quality of sleep declines. This affected my client Denise's ability to sleep comfortably. She wasn't experiencing weight gain or hot flashes, herself, although hot flashes/night sweats can definitely interfere with your ability to sleep.

Experts believe that the **body's capacity to produce enough hormones to support quality sleep becomes limited during and after menopause**, so I worked with Denise on a **new strength-building program** that supported her metabolism and hormone balance. I describe it later in this book.

### 4. Fatigue & Lack of Energy

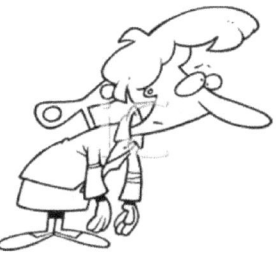

Have you ever felt as though you just didn't have an ounce of energy left?

Susanne used to describe to me how, some days, she ***felt like she couldn't take another step***. That intense fatigue was her enemy when it came to doing the things that she loved, including regular workouts. Stretches of extreme exhaustion often overwhelmed her.

Lisa used to describe an **up-and-down tiredness** during menopause, where she felt good one minute, and then like a truck had hit her, the next.

During menopause, the feeling of *chronic or crushing fatigue is a normal but rather distressing symptom* that can be particularly debilitating.

Susanne and Lisa were like a lot of women who develop a total lack of energy, and who can feel completely exhausted, even if they haven't done a thing. Fatigue can cause total body exhaustion and poor energy levels that aren't relieved just by bed rest. Until some successful remedies are introduced to these sufferers, it can lead to a feeling of helplessness.

Some other common signs of this disorder, beyond exhaustion, include: **depression, irritability, daytime tiredness, lack of concentration, and the need to rest at unusual times.**

There are both *physical and psychological causes* for menopausal fatigue.

I worked with Susanne and Lisa, first, on their hormone balance, and then, on affirmations and coaching, in order to support their motivation to work through it.

The natural menopausal decrease in estrogen and progesterone levels also affects your ***levels of cortisol,*** which is the ***hormone that regulates tiredness***.

***Cortisol levels rise out of control in a body when the amounts of estrogen and progesterone decrease***.

Lack of energy and fatigue are the consequence.

So … here's another reason to maintain hormonal balance during menopause. *To stabilize and possibly avoid crashing and chronic fatigue*. I talk about that in my nutrition plan recommendations, later.

Another factor that contributes to fatigue is when your body's ***adrenal glands become fatigued due to prolonged emotional or financial stress, and/or poor eating habits***.

**Adrenal fatigue** comes about when these critical glands function at a sub-optimal level. They will struggle to meet the high demands of cortisol production, which leads eventually to their depletion.

In addition to tiredness, Lisa complained about *salt cravings, brain fog/absent-mindedness*, and a *decreased sex drive*. These are also symptoms of adrenal fatigue. In working with her, we addressed these by **managing Lisa's hormone balance through nutrition and supplements.**

Susanne's fatigue had a number of psychological causes, including *stress and irritability.*

***I work with all of my clients to alleviate stress from their lives. I share with you my three strongest recommendations for doing this in chapter 5.***

In my experience, Susanne and others who lower their stress and reduce their anxiety as part of a comprehensive lifestyle adjustment during menopause really do lessen the severity of fatigue's most debilitating symptoms.

As I discuss in later chapters, **stress management** in menopause includes: getting a proper amount of sleep; making dietary changes that increase the nutritional value of what you eat; and exercising correctly.

Since hormonal imbalance is the primary cause of menopausal fatigue, women like Lisa and Susanne were also helped tremendously by ***taking some of the natural supplements that I discuss in chapter 7***.

If you still don't getting relief, then you may want to speak to your physician about other forms of hormone therapy.

## 5. Depression and Mood Swings

Menopause doesn't only prompt uncomfortable *physical* symptoms. ***It can also turn a woman´s emotions into an out-of-control pendulum***, and afflict her with ***mood swings.***

More than 50% of my clients have described mood swings as they approached menopause.

Fortunately, there are ways to manage this emotional turbulence.

A **mood swing** is an *extreme fluctuation or drastic shift in your emotional state.*

My client AnnaMaria used to feel like she had emotional reactions to thing that were wildly out of line with whatever had triggered them, or were on a bigger scale than whatever had brought them on. These *swings are directly related to menopausal changes in the hormones* that regulate mood and emotions.

Although moodiness is a super common symptom—up to 75% of all peri-menopausal women report mood swings—many women find the phenomenon very troubling.

Each woman manages her emotions and stress differently, when they arise in her work and home environments. In the same way, *experiences of mood swings in menopause differ from woman to woman*, as well.

AnnaMaria described frequent mood changes and irritability. Another of my clients, Denise, found that she was *emotional about things that she couldn't really explain, logically:* sometimes she would be very impatient, which was unusual for her; at other times she was anxious for no apparent reason.

Other women have described **feeling sad**, more **stressed out** than usual, **aggressive, nervous, melancholy,** and even a **blah emotion** with **low motivation.**

AnnaMaria and Denise first started to feel better about their menopausal mood swings when they brought some awareness to them. As they learned more about the hormone cycle, and how it is impacted by exercise and nutrition, they began to feel better equipped to deal with their emotional reactivity. They also began to treat the underlying causes.

Like all women going into peri-menopause, my clients' key reproductive hormone levels were falling, so they were being *affected by this disturbance in the body's natural equilibrium.* They attuned themselves to this fluctuation in their body's chemical process, as a starting point.

They were also interested to learn about the *role that estrogen plays in the brain's production of* <u>*serotonin*</u>.

You've probably heard how serotonin is called "the mood-regulating neurotransmitter." It turns out that the sensitivity of serotonin receptors in a woman's brain is also affected by her estrogen level.

So, part of a woman's mood swings, depression, and other psychological disturbances during menopause come from *changes in estrogen levels, as they temporarily disturb serotonin production in the brain.*

When I first take on a client like AnnaMaria or Denise, we do a nutrition- and exercise-analysis together. But we also talk about life stressors, and how they are impacting a woman's life outside of the challenges of menopause.

Most of the women that I work with in their 40s and 50s are already *stretched by the stresses of family and work*. When they begin to experience the disruption of hot flashes, the crush of fatigue, and the sleep problems that are so common in peri-menopause, they have described to me how *these symptoms contribute directly to their destabilized mood and emotions*.

I have other clients who, as they experience certain other *uncomfortable physical changes* that are part of the menopause process (like **vaginal dryness,**

**weight gain, and migraines),** find that their mood swings exacerbated, too.

I make **lowering stress** and addressing emotional happiness a big part of my three-part MENOPAUSE SUCCESS TRIANGLE. Stress reduction is *just as critical as are adjustments to food and exercise.*

I'll explain what helped AnnaMaria and Denise with their mood swings later, in chapter 5.

### 6. Brain Fog

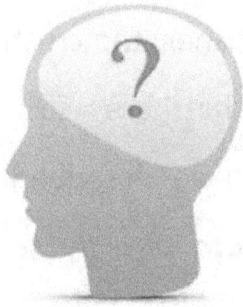

*Brain fog does exist!*

Clients Nadi and Michelle often shook their heads at the start of our workout sessions, complaining about this *mysterious cloud that came over their minds* during menopause. It led them sometimes to forget even the simplest things.

I shared with them the studies that confirm that memory problems—or "brain fog" —are really common during menopause.

Do you suffer from this symptom? Then you know how frustrating it can be to deal with.

Brain fog is more technically known as "cognitive dysfunction," and it describes *a state of mental fuzziness or confusion* that is generally caused by an underlying health issue. **Symptoms** may include:

a) An inability to concentrate or to focus on details
b) A feeling of mental fuzziness or cloudiness
c) A lack of mental clarity
d) An inability to remember things, events, names, or details
e) A decreased attention span
f) Mental fatigue
g) A feeling of being emotionally distanced, or of not caring as much as you normally would, in any given situation

Don't these all sound like menopause symptoms to you?

You and Nadi and Michelle are far from being alone!

Roughly **two-thirds of women complain about forgetfulness or "brain fog" during menopause**.

Nadi would say that she just didn't feel quite right; that she couldn't think as clearly as she used to.

For Michelle, brain fog was really episodic: sometimes she was her usual self, sharp as a tack. Then, on other days, she felt like she had left her entire brain back at the house. She didn't feel present. She had a hard time concentrating on details. And it was as though her focus was shot.

One problem that I found women to have with brain fog was that, as common as it is, *conventional medicine doesn't recognize or diagnose it as an illness or condition*. So, until they began to talk about it with a coach or with other women, Michelle and Nadi felt like they were on their own, and had to suffer in silence.

I've had other clients who were menopausal, but ***didn't think that their brain fog was a symptom!*** They just thought that they were going through some mental decline because of their daily stress, or as an inevitable "sign of aging."

I was really happy to show these women that TWO recent research studies found that **cognitive decline and memory problems associated with menopause are _real_,** and that they may be **linked to fluctuating levels of hormones in the brain.**

One study, at New York's University of Rochester, found that pre- and post-menopausal women aged 40-60 performed worse on tests of memory and cognition during the year after they had had their last period than in any time leading up to the menopause. Researchers also found that, while it is unclear why menopause may affect cognition, hormones are most likely are involved.

"In the months after a woman has her last period, hormonal changes are most abrupt," said senior study researcher Pauline Maki, PhD, Director of Women's Mental Health Research at the University of Illinois in Chicago.

As a woman approaches menopause, her ovaries gradually produce **less estrogen, which is crucial for thinking and remembering.** The good news coming out of this research is that changes in memory associated with menopause appear to be **temporary,** according to their data, and are **not linked to diseases such as dementia and Alzheimer's disease.**

The second study, led by researchers at Brigham and Women's Hospital in Boston, suggests that the younger a woman is when she experiences surgical menopause (which is the removal of her uterus—hysterectomy—and one or both ovaries—

oophorectomy), the faster she will experience declines in her ability to remember times and places. For further details, read about the studies here, at myhealthnewsdaily.com.

### 7. Night Sweats

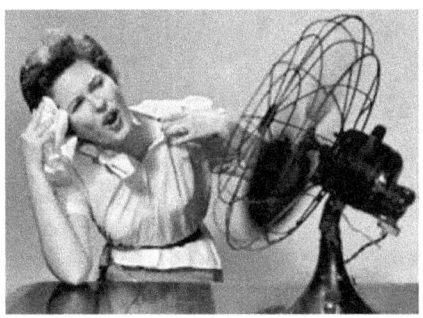

Night sweats used to disturb Deborah's sleep a great deal. And after any night when she had had severe hot flash-type symptoms while sleeping, and when she had woken up in sticky sheets with a pounding heart coated in perspiration and upset, she was naturally a bit fatigued and irritable the next day.

She often found it hard to fall back to sleep after these episodes, too, and noticed that her mood swings were more pronounced after being awoken that way.

Like hot flashes, *night sweats are also brought on by your newly fluctuating levels of key regulating hormones*.

Estrogen is involved, as is the brain area called the **hypothalamus, which regulates temperature**, and which becomes disoriented by variances in estrogen levels.

A key brain chemical called **norepinephrine is another part of the trigger for night sweats, as are brain receptors, sweat glands, and dilating blood vessels** that flood your system with perspiration and blood, and surge your fast-beating heart.

About 80% of women in menopause experience either night sweats or hot flashes, so if you're sharing Deborah's experience, you're not alone.

But in my experience, after *applying some of the natural remedies that I recommend below, only a small percentage of women find their night sweats so*

***extreme that they request medication in order to handle them.***

When I began to work with Deborah and others who wanted to address night sweats that were disturbing their sleep and raising their anxiety, I had each of my clients begin their lifestyle adjustment by checking out the following ideas:

a) *Deep Breathing*: slow, rhythmic breathing, with deep inhalations and extended, complete exhalations have been shown to reduce night sweats, and to help you return to sleep after being awoken by a hot or clammy feeling.

b) *Discovering patterns*: Deborah kept a notepad or journal by her bed, and when night sweats came on (you can do this the next morning, too—just don't forget!), she'd write down things that she had done the evening before. This included what she ate and drank, or whether she had smoked or taken certain medications.

She began to *see patterns emerge* that seemed to *trigger her most uncomfortable night*—for her, they often came on after eating spicy food or drinking red wine.

c) *Keep cool*: Deborah started to keep a fan by her bedside, and opened her window at night. She switched to light-weight sheets, even in winter, and found new night clothes made with natural fibers that had cooling properties. (For some product ideas, see the Resources in Chapter 10.)

d) *Try hormone replacement therapy (HRT)*: Deborah didn't need to go this route, but some women do find that medication addresses the most severe of symptoms. *This is something to discuss with your doctor* if, for some reason, you don't have success with the many natural remedies and lifestyle adjustments that I recommend throughout this book. There are **risks involved with the HRT approach**, as you may have read. I encourage you to **ask for updates** about those when you have conversations with medical practitioners, and be sure that your doctors share with you the most current data from HRT studies.

e) *The natural approach*: There are many supplements that I discuss throughout this book, particularly in chapter 7. Hot flashes/night sweats are some of the first places where Deborah and Lizz noticed relief when they tried herbal supplements like *black cohosh*, and a Chinese herbal remedy called ***dang gui bu xue tang*** that includes dong quai.

f) *Exercise*: Every woman that I work with makes a change to her exercise and activity plan. For some, like Barbara and Lizz, these new fitness regimes helped them to lose weight and manage menopause symptoms. Others, like Denise, didn't have weight issues, but by *increasing their physical activity and cardio-vascular fitness*, they not only felt healthier, but their night sweats tapered off, as well.

~~~~~~~~

If you are in your 40s or 50s, you may have begun to experience physiological changes in addition to these 7 Magic Symptoms that may or may not be peri-menopause. In my resource chapter, I list some books and websites that provide a complete list of symptoms, like "34-Menopause-Symptoms."

There is a broad range of physical, mental, and emotional indicators associated with menopause. They all impact women differently.

What I observe in my practice, unfortunately, is this:

*Many women aren't noticing their symptoms as menopause, or don't yet recognize that they can address them in concrete, productive ways.*

So please, take stock.

Where are you, in this range of changes?

The rest of this book will make clear how to be more comfortable and successful in managing the menopause transition. And it will even give you loads of tips on how to have fun doing it!

# -TWO-

## Top 6 Menopause Myths

OK: everybody has heard *something* about menopause. Maybe from your mom or from your friends or in the media.

The thing is, **plenty of what you hear out there is <u>wrong</u>**! Just plain *Not True*.

I want to *debunk these big misconceptions* right up front, because I think that they hurt women who are ready to manage peri-menopause in a healthy, holistic way.

As you take your first steps towards a successful menopause experience, I believe that you should, and can, build and maintain a **positive, open mindset** based on **solid information.**

So—have you heard any of these?? Let me lay them on you, and then I'll tell you what I know to be true about each of these Top 6 Myths:

1. Menopause is a disease or medical condition.

***Menopause is neither***: it is a natural biological process.

It's not a medical illness.

It's just **the stage in a woman's life when she stops having her monthly period;** it is a **normal part of aging**, and it marks the end of a woman's reproductive years.

That said, there are definitely strategies, medicines, and other treatments available to address some of the symptoms of menopause when they disrupt a woman's life.

My clients have had great success with lifestyle changes and natural remedies, all of which support my conviction that *menopause is not a "medical" condition.* It is a process that can be approached with comfort, grace, and joy.

2. Most of the body changes women experience at midlife are due to menopause.

   **This is half true**.

   Some of a woman's midlife body changes are related to the shifts in hormones that I described in chapter 1, because menstruation is ceasing and the role of your ovaries is changing.

   <u>BUT</u> some of the symptoms that I address in this book are **part of the natural aging process**, and, as they mature, my male clients have to deal with changes in their metabolism and body chemistry, too.

3. Saliva testing is effective for determining if a midlife woman has the "right" levels of hormones.

   Many of my clients—particularly those that I meet in their 40s like Lizz, Lizzette, and AnnaMaria—did **both types of hormone tests** at some point during their peri-menopause.

   One reason: *each test has limitations*.

**Blood tests** are sometimes considered more accurate.

But **complete saliva testing** is taken at four points throughout the day, so it measures more thoroughly the various shifts in your menopause hormone levels.

Saliva and blood both take readings of **estradiol, progesterone, testosterone, DHEA-S,** and **cortisol;** only blood can measure **HGH.** Lizzette liked how convenient the saliva tests were—she could do them herself, at home, on her own time.

*They only showed us levels of free, unbound bio-available hormone molecules*, however, and I know that our body tissues also use free-form and weakly-bound forms of these molecules, as well. Her subsequent blood test picked up on those forms.

I am also concerned about the plastic tubes in home saliva kits—they can degrade your hormones through their own estrogenic compounds. So please *try to use glass tubes* wherever possible.

I also recommend that you **make sure** that the company reading your saliva test is **using hormone assays designed for saliva, not blood;** the incorrect assays will produce flaws.

And also be aware that **common medicines for colds and allergies can interfere with saliva production** and how hormones are excreted into it.

So ... when testing, do both types!

4. Menopause will decrease my mental ability

Lisa, Michelle, and Nadi complained about short-term memory problems and difficulty concentrating sometimes, as I mentioned. Occasionally, they even felt disoriented.

**Everyone misplaces their keys from time to time**: it may not even be menopause-related, and it's highly unlike that it's early onset dementia, either!

These women soon understood how the **changing estrogen levels found in peri-menopausal women contributed to their own forgetfulness, and even their** *spaciness*. Cognitive function is regulated by various neurotransmitters which affect both concentration and memory; these are produced in part by estrogen.

So, these women discovered how **variations in their estrogen levels were affecting the flow of blood to their brains,** making them feel mental confusion or occasional dizziness and disorientation.

That said, Nadi can already attest to the fact that, after menopause, many of her symptoms ceased. I have a few other clients who elected to supplement their lifestyle and nutrition changes with bio-identical estrogen in order to support their mental clarity.

Michelle exercised her concentration during menopause by stretching and challenging her mind, like a muscle. She loves doing puzzles, and even started to learn a new language. You can try taking up a musical instrument, reading more books, or learning different types of dance or sports that require memorization of mental patterns and routines.

### 5. Menopausal women are not sexy

Women are still *as sexy as they feel,* no matter their age or biological stage.

That said, Mother Nature did build in a natural increase in sexual desire around ovulation. So, when that event cycle of menstruation/ovulation ceases during menopause, *women won't feel the same monthly "boost" in their sex drive*.

Lower levels of estrogen affected Denise's sexuality. She always found that it used to **elevate her mood ...** both in the brain and the genitals. Without it flowing through her system, she experienced *vaginal dryness* which made sex uncomfortable and much less pleasurable.

When Nadi got her blood tests back (which she ordered for us to develop a hormone-balancing nutrition plan for her), she found that she had **very low levels of the male hormone *testosterone***, which plays a part in a woman's sex drive.

Like most women, before menopause, Nadi's system only had a small amount of testosterone, anyway. But now, its level in her body had dropped to below normal, as a result of her natural aging process. She began to take tiny doses of bio-identical testosterone cream, and soon returned to feeling like her own sexual self.

My client Lizzette found that both localized estrogen cream and topical vitamin E oil were solutions that helped her out. Some women find that the **SSRIs** that they take for mild depression also *suppress their libido.* Experimenting with alternative medications can change your feelings markedly.

All that said, ***women stay sexy by having sex***, and by finding ways to support and enjoy it.

Some postmenopausal women tell me that they *now have a greater sex drive than ten years ago*: they're free of any anxieties about pregnancy, and they have fewer responsibilities for their grown children.

I think that by first *staying fit so that you feel physically great,* then by *supporting yourself with vaginal lubricants and, possibly, some supplements*, you can really counter this myth.

6. Menopause makes you gain weight:
   "Menopause has done me in ... I'll never get my body back."

Barbara said that to me.

**But "never" was an exaggeration, once she learned about** the menopause metabolism.

I devote the entire next chapter to that. And to how **your metabolism,** like Barbara's and everyone else's, is **definitely different with age**.

But the fact that hits this myth head-on is this: really, **it's poor diet, lack of exercise, and shifts in metabolism that lead to weight gain, not menopause per se**.

For Barbara, I helped her to put together *a balanced diet* plus *a tailored activity plan* that brought her back to a **good, healthy weight**, while she *revved up her metabolism with more lean muscle.*

The added benefit to Barbara's accomplishments was is that she was able to ***reduce her risk of heart attack and stroke by lowering her blood cholesterol levels***. Down went her ***risks for other metabolic syndromes like insulin resistance***, too.

I'm confident that **you won't let menopause "do you in," either.** You can reclaim a fit, trim body plus keep your muscles and joints strong, while you lower your risk of osteoporosis, at the same time.

~~~~~~~~~~

So, ***put these myths aside.***

Let's **get real about your metabolism** in detail.

Then, we'll dive in to the Menopause Success Triangle, and how to make it work for ***you***.

# -THREE-

## The Menopause Metabolism

I've told you about Lizzette, Jillian, and Barbara. They had each **gained 15-30 pounds** in the face of their changing menopause metabolism.

Through **lifestyle adjustments and supplements**, they were successful in reversing this trend and in dropping many dress sizes.

I think that **their progress to success** began when they <u>understood their own menopause metabolism</u> clearly. They recognized **what needed to be different about what and how they ate,** during this new stage of their lives.

**Every great change starts in the mind,** so I want to share with you what I explained to them.

**Here's how you can use that information to** *approach menopause in a different way*.

As we age, our metabolism slows down and we burn fewer calories. This is *mainly because of our reduced muscle mass*.

As we age, our **muscle mass decreases**, and is **replaced with stored fat**. Muscles are more metabolically demanding, and they burn more calories than fat, so a cycle begins. Women like Jillian and Lizzette suddenly **find extra pounds around their hips and belly that they hate**.

I started my coaching sessions with them by letting them know that their **experiences were very normal.** They had *the same changes in and depletion of hormones* that I discussed in chapter 1.

Jillian kept saying that she hadn't been eating any differently; **maybe even eating less.** Still, she found that she was changing shape and size.

Totally understandable.

I'll describe the alterations that she decided to make in what and how she ate, once I *armed her with this additional information.*

**Hormones** like estrogen, progesterone, testosterone, and androgen directly **impact** not just your moods and interior thermostat, but *your metabolism and fat storage*, as well. *When they fluctuate, so does your success at weight control* through traditional eating and exercise strategies.

For example, when your ovaries create less *ESTROGEN*, your peri-menopausal body will *try to replace it by building up fat cells that can also produce estrogen*. Then, your body literally tries to convert any calories that you eat into fat, just so that you have more estrogen-producers.

As your *PROGESTERONE* levels fall, your body sometimes *bloats or retains water*, and that feels like weight gain, too, and affects how your clothes fit.

The dip in **TESTOSTERONE** that Nadi found in her blood test explained the *challenge* that she was having in *creating lean muscle mass out of ingested calories.* Because muscle burns more calories than fat, her lowered *testosterone* meant that she was *building less muscle*, which was contributing to her lower metabolism because her *calories were burning more slowly*.

I gave her plenty of exercises and diet tips to rebuild that muscle in order to turn around her weight gain.

The last piece of information for you to know about hormones and metabolism is that *one of them actually increases* during menopause: **ANDROGEN.** This hormone is responsible for the *redistribution of fat from curvy, pear-shaped hips straight to your belly and abdomen.* As you probably know, this is *a more dangerous spot for anyone to have fat.* I'll talk about **belly-fat exercises** that had huge impact on most every woman I coach.

There are a *few other things that you should know* about, too, that affect menopausal metabolism and weight gain.

One is **INSULIN RESISTANCE.** This is particularly challenging *if you subscribe to a high-carbohydrate, low-fat diet.* After age 40 or 50, many of us develop some version of insulin resistance. The *body turns all of our carbohydrate calories into fat*, instead of dividing it between fat, muscle, and other byproducts. **Processed foods, as well as white flour/white rice/white sugar/white potatoes,** and **high fructose corn syrup** are culprits that have been linked to this syndrome, in addition to the natural aging cycle.

Barbara and Jillian adapted beautifully to the menopause diet suggestions in chapter 6, once I challenged them to *radically shift their diet away from simple, refined carbohydrates*.

Deborah, on the other hand, *attributed her menopausal weight gain to* STRESS.

That is why de-stressing is a core tenet of my three-part Menopause Success Triangle, outlined in detail in chapter 5.

I explained to Deborah that *the hormones that circulate in a stressed-out body tell her metabolism to store fat rather than to burn it off*, so part of our work together was to help her body chill out that particular reaction.

The last thing that you need to analyze, in order to understand your own menopause metabolism, is **GENETICS.**

Yes, they also *play a role in weight gain* during and after menopause.

Cristi and Rae were sisters that I worked with. Their parents tended to gain weight in the abdomen. This increased the likelihood that they would, as well.

I'm sorry about that: *genes aren't something that you can change,* at this point!

BUT there are <u>**plenty of ways to lessen the impact of your genetics**</u>.

My client Michelle had no issues with weight gain during menopause, but she did begin to notice *thigh and hip cellulite,* which is a fat deposit visible under the layer of the skin.

This is **another development** that comes with age. It correlates to what *can be occurring inside* of a woman's body, like a **thickening of the artery walls** that increase a woman's **chance of cardiac arrest**.

Here's what worked for Jillian and Cristi, Michelle and Deborah, as they addressed the challenges of the menopause metabolism: they implemented the many lifestyle strategies that I lay out in the next few chapters.

The Menopause Success Triangle.

And **the best thing that they did** to minimize this and other menopause symptoms was *to develop their appreciation for the fact that they were on a positive, natural journey.*

This trip **definitely looked different than their reproductive stage of life**, but it **wasn't necessarily better or worse.**

For example, these women came to appreciate the corollary fact that *a little weight gain in midlife does protect your hips* and other vital structural bones from osteoporosis and breaking, while it *also prepares you to combat other illnesses*.

Some fat **even eases anxiety and hot flashes**, if you can believe it!

So, I'm going to share all of the strategies for weight loss and metabolism success that worked for them, but please remember: **not fitting into old clothes is not the end of your world.**

~~~~~~~~

The **secret to preventing weight gain** is the same for all ages: *consume fewer calories than you burn*.

During menopause, Michelle and Jillian found that they *had to work harder to apply this formula*, while they had to *find natural ways to* support their rate of calorie burn by *revving up their metabolism*. But they could do it. They *did* do it.

**Let me tell YOU how they did it.**

# -FOUR-

## Motivation & Mindset

As they hit peri-menopause, my clients Denise and Lizzette found that they **began to lose some of their vitality**. They couldn't maintain their previous health and fitness routines, either.

These women asked me whether or not this feeling was inevitable, now that they were in menopause, along with the weight gain, loss of muscle tone, and less energy that they were experiencing.

**My answer to them was, NO.**

But before we developed their new exercise and nutrition plans, I showed them how **the path to creating a successful, positive menopause experience** *began in their MINDS.*

I believe that my **strategies for improving motivation and mindset** can *help someone at any time* in their lives.

As Denise and Lizzette began the process of peri-menopause, they learned *how critical their mindsets were to boosting their personal motivation,* and *to establishing a routine that inspired a positive, generous, forward-looking attitude,* and that enhanced all aspects of their wellbeing.

Lack of motivation was the toughest problem that Denise had to deal with. She found that every other change in her body could be managed gracefully once she had **the motivation to learn about and implement healthier options**. Until she did, though, she felt **lethargic** about any attempt to improve her situation.

I had another client whose **lack of motivation was the root cause of her menopausal depression**.

What I shared with Denise and Lizzette is that there are **three components for developing an ideal menopausal mindset:**

▶ Belief Systems
▶ Affirmations
▶ Goal Setting

Together, they **work to motivate** someone to establish the lifestyle changes that I describe in the next few chapters.

*Once any woman embraces these three ideas, they find it so much easier to adopt new fitness and nutrition regimes.*

**THEN**, they can experience menopause in **an entirely different way.**

## 1. BELIEF SYSTEMS

Lizzette's successful menopause experience began the moment that she *overcame the feeling* that she had *to accept the negative effects* of what she was going through.

Once she rid herself of the idea that menopause was a disease, *she didn't feel like it was "something that was happening to her."*

The fact is that it is just *an* experience: a **natural, normal one that you can direct and co-create in concrete ways**.

In order to develop your own happy, healthy menopause life, you first need to shift your thinking.

You need to be willing to say that *what you are going through is OK*.

That you **accept it.**

That you **embrace it.**

That you are even *looking forward to it*.

Because this is *merely a new stage in life*, one that you are willing to be excited about.

Lizzette decided that she was going to lose her "doom and gloom" attitude about menopause. She started to see it instead as something fantastic, exciting, and new.

She needed to *make this PARADIGM SHIFT*, to activate her own success.

I encourage you to do the same.

You are entering the **second stage of your life.**

*What you experienced during your reproductive years was just the first chapter.*

*Now, you are moving on to chapter two.*

*What are you going to do to make <u>this</u> part <u>better</u> than the first?*

## 2. AFFIRMATIONS

Doing affirmations is *the daily practice of cultivating positivity, vision, and well-being*.

Denise found that **affirmations were the key to reprogramming her mental state**, and to **rewiring her mental hard-drive in order to build a happier life.**

Affirmations are particularly important during menopause because many women like Denise have been <u>*told certain things*</u> *that contribute to their confusion, weakness, or inability to move forward* with enthusiasm and good health.

Myself, I've used affirmations in order to **overcome my own personal disabilities and challenges**.

I encourage you **to make them part of your daily routine.**

Affirmations are **powerful mini-messages** that keep Denise and others like her moving forward.

The first thing that Denise did was to **<u>find a list of affirmations that moved her, personally.</u>** She wrote and researched her own sayings, messages, and inspirational words. In addition, she also borrowed some ideas from **my list of personal favorites**, which I share below.

You can **start today by collecting words and phrases that make you feel EMPOWERED.**

I asked Denise and Lizzette both to **affirm daily their reasons for wanting to be HEALTHY and STRONG**. Doing this has helped them to stay positive.

On days that they were tempted to go back to their old ways of eating, for example, they reminded themselves **that they deserved better**.

You can do the same. ***You, too, have the power to influence your menopausal symptoms***.

One of my favorite affirmations is this, by the great Tony Robbins:

"Every day in every way I'm getting better and better."

Another wonderful reminder, one that I use at the end of my coaching sessions and interactions, is this:

"Stay Active. Stay Positive. Embrace your beauty."

Add those words to your personal list, if you'd like.

Or:

"Today I accept these challenges so that tomorrow will be better."

## 10 Affirmations for Menopause Success

1. Today I celebrate my beauty, strength, and inner peace.
2. Get up, Get going, and Get over it.
3. I am grateful for all that I am, for all that I have, and for all that I experience.
4. I love and accept myself just as I am.
5. I let go of blame and I speak my truth authentically—without judging myself or others.
6. Today I empower myself to embrace my power and stand strong in the face of all challenges.
7. Menopause ... What?
8. I accept the CHANGES IN MY LIFE and embrace the future.
9. My mind and body are healthy and strong, and I nourish them with my spirit which is POWERED BY MY FAITH.
10. I am... (Fill in the blank—e.g. I am *powerful*, I am *grateful*, I am *beautiful*.)

## 3. GOAL *ACHIEVING*

I've always been *a goal-setting person*.

At a young age, I learned about **the power of focused effort to reach specific goals.**

Goal setting is important, but only as the first step to success. Lots of people teach goal setting, but not many experts also go on to share the specific ways that you achieve those goals.

Let me ask you a few questions. How would you answer them?

▶ What makes me happy?

▶ Do I currently like how I see myself in the mirror?

▶ Am I living my ideal life?

▶ What challenges do I see getting in the way of me attaining my goals, and of my creating a healthy, happy menopause life?

I want you to think about these as I give you my 5-Step Goal-Setting for Menopause Formula.

This formula is *guaranteed to help you navigate through the landmines of menopause confusion*!!

Once you learn **not just to set goals,** but also how to *achieve* them, your success at anything that you undertake will go through the roof.

This formula works great on health and fitness goals.

I'm going to tell you about Michelle, and how we *followed the following five steps to realize her weight-loss and stress-reduction goals*.

But I use this approach in **ALL ASPECTS** *of my life*.

It works for **setting and attaining financial and career goals.**

For **personal growth and spiritual goals.**

Even **fun goals,** as well!

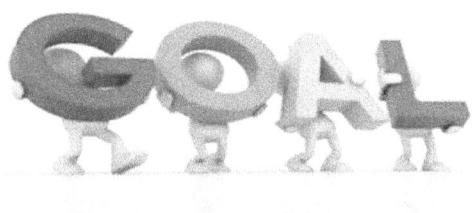

## 5 Simple Steps to Achieving any Menopause Goal

1.  **DECIDE:**

First, you need to decide ___specifically___ **what it is that you want.** And ___when___ **you want to do it** by.

**Goals** need a ___date___ in order to be achieved.

So, for example, let's say that **your first health goal is to lose 30 pounds in 3 months**.

That is <u>very concrete,</u> which is essential to the goal-setting and -attaining process.

Then, as part of your deciding process, you can **break this goal into** milestones.

So, target 10 pounds of weight-loss each month, or 2-1/2 pounds each week.

**This specificity is KEY** to your success.

Remember: goal-setting is wasted effort without goal-achieving.

## 2. PLAN:

Next, *reverse engineer* your goal.

Think through *each step of the process* from here to your target, **including each of the milestones** that you laid out in step 1.

Design the framework needed for each step in order to accomplish your goal.

For me, this involves *creating a checklist of all the tasks necessary* to reach a specific result.

So, **how, specifically, can you achieve this goal of losing 30 pounds in 3 months**?

Well, here you would *identify a workout strategy that supports losing that 2-1/2 pounds each week*. It would include a weekly regime of 3 days of cardio training, 3 days of strength training, and 1 day of relaxation and walking.

Once you implement that concrete plan, you will have a better path to achieve your end result.

### 3. TAKE IMMEDIATE ACTION:

***Do it now.***

**IMMEDIATELY.**

***DON'T WAIT!!***

Once you have a plan in place, ***take your first steps*** towards actualizing it ***right away***.

Part of your planning may involve reverse engineering a way to succeed on those steps.

For example, if you adopt the strategy above, but are not yet a member of a gym or working out with a coach, you need to enlist a workout buddy **The Next Day**.

Also, **write your goals down and put them in a place that you see *all the time.***

On your bathroom mirror.

Above the car radio.

On the refrigerator door.

Be sure that this is *a place you visit often*, so that you can reinforce these ideas. Be sure to let your goals sink into your long-term thinking by viewing—and reviewing them—regularly. Read them aloud daily, too.

**The Action step is super important, because *action helps you to create the belief systems that are essential for breaking through any self-doubt*, or overcoming any negative feelings.**

***Doing creates motion*, and that then creates positive, forward-looking emotions.**

### 4. MEASURE/TRACK YOUR PROGRESS:

This step is *my secret sauce.*

Measuring each task as you complete it gives you **reference points that indicate how close you are to achieving your goals**.

**Setting solid milestones** is simple: after you frame-work your plan and make it clear and specific, *then break it into bite-sized chucks*. Each chunk is a small task that, once completed, adds up and accumulates to manifest your completed goals.

**Anything that we want to achieve has to be _measured._** So, design the way to *put concrete measurement or numbers to your goals* and milestones.

- Maybe it is by **pounds lost** on your home scale
- Maybe it is by **inches melting away** from your waistline, measured with a tape measure at regular intervals.
- Or a calculation of your **body fat ratio**
- Maybe you have a **spiritual goal** (e.g. reading 15 minutes of personal growth material each day), and can **mark off your readings daily** on a bold wall calendar.

*Establish your benchmarks.*

Is your goal **financial**? Use weekly budget reports to note income relative to expenses.

Do you need to save $5,000 by the end of the year? Divvy that up into monthly and weekly milestones, and keep a checklist for each $96 that you put away.

Measuring **fun goals** can be more challenging, but find benchmarks that match your dream.

Say, for example, **you want an all-expenses-paid vacation and it costs $1,000**. Use the goal-attaining formula to set aside a third of the amount each month for three months, then *GO HAVE FUN*!

5.     REWARD YOUR ACHIEVING MILESTONES:

I've always taught my clients that **rewarding yourself is a positive way to reinforce** the fact that you are on your way to achieving your goals.

This has worked super well for my weight-loss and fitness clients. **Create small rewards that are pegged to  achieving each milestone**.

It can be something as small as celebrating with a coffee from Starbucks.

Or purchasing a new pair of sneakers for running.

Your **reward is up to you**, but the key is that you *never reward yourself until you have completed the specific milestone* for that reward.

While attaining your goal of losing 30 pounds after 3 months is a huge success, by itself, still, **you need to plan for ways that you'll reward yourself when you reach your 10- and 20-pound loss marks, too.**

Have you designed a plan to read inspirational material nightly for 90 days? Set a reward once you check 30 days off of your calendar, and after 60 days, too!

And if weight-loss is one of your goals, be sure that you **plan for a maintenance program** to follow up on your success: part of your reward is to keep off all of those pounds that you've shed!

~~~~~~~~

That's the **5-Step Goal-setting for Menopause Formula**.

This formula has helped me:

▶ **Get through college courses**

▶ **Finish weight loss challenges**

▶ **Launch the My Menopause Fix Blog**

It is **simple** and it **works**, but <u>***only if you put the steps into action***</u> in order to achieve the goals that you set.

I bring this formula to all of my clients, and include it in my coaching.

When Michelle came to work with me, for example, she was **49 years old**, **single**, and had a **high level of stress** as she **juggled two demanding jobs**.

Together we developed a **3-part set of goals** that focused on her **desired weight loss**, **improved nutrition**, and **reduced stress**.

First, in order to meet her **goal of losing 30 pounds**, we agreed upon a ***6-month plan***, one that was not overly aggressive because we wanted to minimize her stress and emphasize her achievements.

Michelle complimented her weight loss with a **nutrition goal of eating 4 Paleo-based meals each day** during those 6 months, and to make one of those meals be a liquid protein shake. Prior to setting that goal, she had a propensity to skip meals, and to lack proper daily hydration.

Part of her health and nutrition goals included a *commitment to drink at least 72 ounces water with lemon* each day, and to *walk for 30 minutes on at least 3 days every week.*

In order to achieve her **goal of reducing stress,** Michelle committed to *making her walks a time for relaxation and moving meditation*. She decided to focus only on *relaxing music and breathing* for those 90 minutes every week, and not let her mind drift over to her life's challenges. So there were *no bill payments* *on her mind, or family issues*: her walks were just for breathing and relaxing.

Michelle also wanted to **reprogram her thinking** so that she had **a more positive outlook**, and banished her negative thoughts. So she committed ***to read or listen to an inspirational story or motivational speaker for 15 minutes every day,**** as well. This served as an affirmation of her personal-growth, and reinforced her positive mindset.

~~~~~~~~

You know how strongly I believe that *having a positive mindset is the **TRUE SECRET** to* The Menopause Success Triangle.

Achieving the goals that you set is going to *make your spirits soar.* And show you the *great power of your mind to create a healthy, happy menopause experience*.

Goal setting is a **process** and a **skill.**

You improve by doing it **often** and **consistently**.

So I encourage you to TAKE ACTION TODAY!

Here's my challenge to you:

**Write down a list of 12 goals. TODAY. Select 3 health & fitness goals, 3 financial goals, 3 spiritual or personal growth goals, and 3 fun goals!**

**Write them: *don't just think them*.**

Then, *put them where you can see them.*

Choose a spot where you are sure to read them at least twice each day.

**<u>Make the practice of affirming your goals become part of your daily habits.</u>**

This is an important aspect of goal-attainment: keep your goals at the forefront of your mind, so that you don't forget about them.

Of course, when you begin your goal-setting and goal-planning, you are fired up and motivated. But, as days and weeks go by, life can get in the way of our goals. We can begin to feel less inspired.

*But when you <u>see</u> your goals every day, you maintain focus.*

So … **make your goals.**

**Be specific.**

**Break them down into attainable milestones and tasks.**

Then, each time you hit a target, **reward yourself and have a blast!**

~~~~~~~~

Remember: *menopause is not a chronic disease that takes away from you everything pleasant about life*.

Start to <u>shift your mental paradigm</u>!

Stop treating menopause as a problem.

Continue to affirm it as a <u>natural process</u>, *not the sad end* of something precious.

The fact of the matter is, menopause can mark *the significant beginning* of a more health-conscious life for you.

Like the Roman philosopher Seneca once said:

"Every new beginning comes from some other beginning's new end."

The next time that you suffer from menopause "lack of motivation," tell yourself that *there is a remedy just around the corner.*

I empower you to **step out of your comfort zone**. Implement the Menopause Success Triangle that I outline in the next chapter!

# -FIVE-

## My New Solution:
# The MENOPAUSE SUCCESS TRIANGLE

Lizz was 49 years old when she first saw me speak at an event. After hearing me talk, she checked out my boot camp. Those were her initial steps towards getting her menopause symptoms under control.

Lizz was a woman who had never really worked out as part of her busy life. She walked me through the problems that she was having:

> ▶ **Belly fat**
> ▶ **High cortisol levels**
> ▶ **Hot flashes**
> ▶ **Brain fog**

I shared with her the information from chapter 1 about **her hormones,** so that she could **really visualize what was going on with her metabolism and the physiological changes that she was experiencing**.

She became an amazing client who embraced all three aspects of my Menopause Success Triangle. She *created a whole new menopause experience* for herself.

When we adapted the three parts of this program for Lizz's body and metabolism:

- ▶ **Within 12 weeks, she had lost 14 pounds**
- ▶ **She did a 180-degree turnaround on her eating**
- ▶ **She implemented such a healthy lifestyle that she felt great**
- ▶ **Other women were inspired all around her to try this same system for bringing menopause symptoms under control**

I didn't have the pleasure of knowing Lizz when her first signs of menopause manifested, including her initial weight gain.

*But I wish I had*.

**ANY POINT** in your peri-menopause period is ideal to make these three life-style changes, but *the sooner you do it, the better.*

*Every menopausal woman that I know <u>feels better</u> after*:

- Adapting her eating patterns
- Becoming more physically active, and
- De-stressing

I designed my MENOPAUSE SUCCESS PLAN for Lizz and my many other clients based on **these three legs**.

Then, I tune the plan in response to **each woman's specific body issues and blood tests.**

My ideas, techniques, and strategies worked for Lizz, for Jillian, for Barbara, Nadi, and many others.

In fact, **they've worked for hundreds and hundreds of women aged 42-60** who present some or all of the 34 menopause symptoms.

**THIS IS MY PROMISE:** <u>these are the answers to your menopause prayers!</u>

- ▶ HOW TO EAT HEALTHIER
- ▶ HOW TO TARGET YOUR EXERCISE
- ▶ HOW TO REDUCE STRESS

Then, **you too can put this** *three-cornered stool for success into your menopause life*.

Come on: watch your life become **joyous, beautiful**, and **positive!**

## 1. NUTRITION

**You need to start where I always start:** with a **NUTRITIONAL ANALYSIS.**

**WHY?**

It's the **only way to make this work for you.**

When I begin working with a client, together we look at:

▶ **What she is eating,** and
▶ **What she** *should* **be eating** in order to increase her energy and address any weight gain.

Do you remember my wonderful client, Lizz?

Let me tell you about **how I made this nutrition portion of the SUCCESS TRIANGLE unlock the truths that she needed to succeed.**

Lizz had a hard time understanding how to make the **MACRONUTRIENT BREAKDOWN** in her diet work better for her.

**What's That!?**

Well, **an incorrect balance of <u>protein</u>, <u>fats</u>, and <u>carbohydrates</u> works against the hormonal changes** that always accompany menopause.

**What does That MEAN!?**

For Lizz—and probably for you, too—an incorrect macronutrient balance **exacerbated her symptoms** like **low stamina** and **hot flashes**.

**SO … FIRST WE HAVE TO UNDERSTAND, AND THEN WE HAVE TO ADJUST FOR THIS IMBALANCE.**

From my perspective, women at this stage of life are generally **getting far too little protein to support proper hormone balance. PLUS** their **fats are coming from animals or saturated-fat sources**.

Lizz *needed to add more "good" fats to her diet instead:* nuts, seeds, olive and coconut oil.

AND the *quality of her carbohydrates was having a huge impact on her metabolism*.

Processed foods and refined sugars or grains were contributing to her **INSULIN RESISTANCE,** and making her gain weight.

She needed to *eat many more complex carbs like vegetables and fruit* in order to bring her metabolism back into balance.

Lizz and Barbara were also struggling with **weight gain.**

They needed to understand that *essential nutrients in their diets are not limited to vitamins and minerals*.

I showed them how their *diet broke down by the MAJOR MACRONUTRIENTS:*

> ▶ Protein
> ▶ Carbohydrates
> ▶ Fats

In order to improve their nutritional health and general well-being, I wanted their *macronutrient distribution range to maximize energy, support metabolism, and minimize negative menopause systems.*

## LET'S FIGURE OUT THIS MACRONUTRIENT BALANCE FOR MENOPAUSE...

Each person's body needs a different macronutrient balance, but I find that my menopausal clients respond to one of these three phases:

*A. 40% Carbohydrates-35% Protein-25% Fats:* I call this the Balance Phase. It **supports higher energy, weight reduction**, and the **building of lean muscle** to improve metabolism.

*B. 30% Carbohydrates-20% Protein-50% Fats*: This diet has a **higher fat ratio,** but these are **healthy fats.** This particular diet **contributes to losing belly fat and also supports weight loss**. Healthy fats are nuts, avocados and seeds, **plus** olive oil that has been cold-pressed and stored exclusively in dark glass. (This careful treatment of olive oil prevents oxidation and preserves the oil's beneficial polyphenol compounds, which are the ones that protect your cells, that support anti-inflammation, and that have recently been shown to improve memory!)

Fatty fish and coconut oil are also healthy fats, sometimes called *MUFA*s (mono-unsaturated fats). Together they can **lower the "bad" cholesterol in your body** and **regulate your insulin levels** when you consume carbohydrates.

Like all of my nutrition plans, this one avoids canola and safflower oil wherever possible.

*C. 50% Carbohydrates-30% Protein-20% Fat:* Some of my clients like Nadi and Cristi **need a lower-fat nutritional plan** because they have symptoms like **high blood pressure or higher body fat**. There are plenty of meal plans to accommodate this strategy; after these clients' blood pressure came under control through diet, exercise, and meditation, I then shifted them to the Balance Phase macronutrient diet.

Barbara and Nadi **shed unwanted pounds but never felt hungry** because they followed my recommendation about including protein in each of their many small, frequent meals.

They also learned how important it is to **eat the right <u>amount</u> and the right <u>kind</u> of protein**, as well, so that they got the maximum health benefits possible. Each of their meals or snacks included something off of this list of Good Sources of Protein:

- *Seafood:* Fishes like salmon and tilapia are good sources of protein because they are low in fat. Although salmon is higher in fat, it is an Omega-3/heart-healthy food
- *Chicken or White-Meat Poultry* are lean protein. Avoid dark meat and skin, as they are more saturated with fat. Broil or grill chicken for best diet and nutrition results.
- *Eggs* are one of the least expensive forms of protein. The American Heart Association says that normal healthy adults can safely enjoy an egg a day.

- *Soy*: Fifty grams of soy protein daily can help to lower cholesterol about 3%, plus help to relieve menopausal symptoms such as hot flashes, night sweats, and the heat rage within.
- *Beans* are loaded with fiber and help to keep you feeling full. One half cup is all you need.

I had to strongly encourage Liz and Barbara to *include protein in their* breakfasts.

**Eat a source of protein in the morning like an egg or Greek yogurt, along with a high-fiber grain like whole wheat toast. They help you to feel full longer, and to eat less throughout the day.**

Lizz is always running around on a tight schedule, so I suggested that she have on hand some **Protein-on-the-Go sources**, like a meal replacement drink, cereal/grain bar, or energy bar. Each one should contain *at least six grams of protein.*

For each of my clients, I work up a model meal plan that is based on:

▶ Their optimal macronutrient balance
▶ Their personal tastes

▶ Any allergies

▶ A daily target caloric intake for their initial training period

You might need 1,200 calories. You might find that 1,600 calories is ideal.

You **don't need to micromanage your daily macronutrient levels**, once you are aware of them. With some attention, **you can arrive at a balance** over the week or the month.

I hope that you will *incorporate these ideas* into your own new nutrition and eating strategy. They **work together with the exercise and stress reduction** techniques below.

## WHAT SHOULD MY CALORIE INTAKE BE, THEN?

Before organizing your own daily nutrition strategy, use this interactive weight loss calculator, at free-online-calculator-use.com/healthy-weight-calculator. Calculate how to reach your ideal weight.

Then, **start to think about *strategic nutrition.***

**STRATEGIC NUTRITION is the process of knowing what to eat, when to eat it, why you're eating it, and how much of it to eat**.

Nutrition makes up *70% of the FAT-LOSS MATRIX.* So, it is imperative that you understand this component of the MENOPAUSE SUCCESS TRIANGLE, particularly if fat loss is part of your goal.

When designing your nutrition plan, *you need to know* <u>*what*</u> *to eat* to achieve your specific goals.

For example, *how lean and defined do you want your midsection?* If you want it super tight and toned, you must **strive to lower your body fat** percentage.

I am a strong advocate of CARB CYCLING. This is a *method for systematically changing your carb intake* <u>*each day,*</u> and then *coordinating your carb intake level with specific your activities* for the day.

For example, **on a *HIIT workout day*** (I'll describe that in section 2, below), you might want to *deplete your carb storage in order to really burn some fat*. So, on this day, you would keep your carbohydrate intake fairly low.

I've used this method with many of my private coaching clients, and ***the results are mind blowing***. **You trick your body so that you never totally live without carbs,** but at the same time you don't store any fat.

Sample Carb Cycle, Broken Down By the Day

Let me share with you *one strategy for a 5-day method*. I gave this to Barbara when we were in the *most intense parts of our* weight-loss macronutrient manipulation cycle.

DAY 1: *150 grams*

DAY 2: *125 grams*

DAY 3: *100 grams*

DAY 4: *75 grams*

DAY 5: *50 grams … (your lowest day)*

DAY 6: *Repeat Day 1*

DAY 7: *Repeat Day 2, etc.*

What is GREAT about this—why the 5-day Carb Cycle REALLY works—is because your energy levels stay HIGH, and women never feel like their allowed amounts of carbohydrates are too low on any given day.

SURE: DAY 5 <u>is</u> low … and you may feel a little tired that day. BUT … *you'll feel GREAT the next day, when your carbs storage is boosted back up!*

You can repeat the *5-day Carb Cycle* until you reach your target weight … *or, FOREVER!* ☺ If that fits your lifestyle, of course.

## HOW DO I CALCULATE MY CALORIES FOR THE DAY, THEN?

You want to **divide** the *total number of carb grams* into your *total number of meals,* on any given day.

Some of your meals may have a few more grams than others. But, at the end of the day, *you MUST stay within the total grams FOR THAT DAY.*

Here's something that helped me:

**There are 4 calories/gram of carbs**

**So … 150 grams of carbs=600 total calories**

**On a day when you are allowed 150 grams of carbs—Day 1: 600 of your calories that day would come from carbs.**

Here's some other info for your calculations:

**FAT=9 calories/gram**

**PROTEIN=4 calories/gram**

Now, *I scheduled Barbara's* <u>*workouts*</u> *based around her Carb Cycling.*

Read the next section, on exercise, and this will make sense. But, basically, *on Barbara's heavy Strategic MRT days, I had her consume higher carbs and lower fat*. This really helped her to keep a tight, toned midsection and *never go into a* ketosis state. (**Ketosis** is when your carbohydrate consumption drops too low for too many days; your body senses starvation, and doesn't much like this condition!)

## HOW ABOUT <u>WHEN</u> TO EAT!?

Yes, the "***When to Eat***" part of your Menopause Success Triangle Nutrition Plan is ***just as important as*** <u>**what**</u> **to eat.**

Clients like Lizzette and Lisa <u>struggled</u> to ***achieve their goals of a* flat belly**. They had tried diets and exercise programs, but they ***couldn't attain a sexier, toned, defined, midsection.***

I coached them on ***when to consume calories***, as well as ***when NOT to***.

This nutritional strategy is a little more complex than just not eating carbs after 7pm, or having protein after a workout. But, even though knowing when to eat your calories is a science, my menopausal clients have become masters at it.

***And many of them now have ridiculous abs to show for it!***

Once you lock in to a macronutrient balance and caloric target, plan your meals out for every 3 hours.

*Begin with the start of your day,* and *measure them until you go to bed.*

Don't go to bed starving, but don't eat a heavy high-fat meal right before bed, either.

*I don't believe in the myth that it is unhealthy to eat after a certain time.* If you don't go to sleep early, or if you work at night, feel free to plan your meals according to your own unique lifestyle.

I do believe that you should **start your day with a hearty, balanced breakfast,** followed by a **moderate calorie snack, lunch, low-fat/low-carb shake, dinner,** and **evening snack.**

OKAY, SO … WHAT DO I EAT?!?!

**WHAT TO EAT** is the *biggest question that I receive* from my clients when it comes to flattening out the midsection.

Just like menopause, there are *many myths and lies* circulating around this topic. Women are *confused about what to eat* in order to affect those *key menopause symptoms:* **weight-gain** and **belly fat**.

Chapter 6 is my **PERFECT MENOPAUSE DIET.**

That's there for an important reason!

I have found that the *Paleo Diet strategy* is the <u>**most successful for achieving hormonal balance, high energy, weight loss, and flat bellies.**</u>

In general, at each meal, your plate should have a portion of veggies, lean meat, fibrous greens, and grains.

My clients *love this idea of dividing their plate*!

It's really a simple rule that has made Lizzette's, Barbara's, and Lisa's lives *so much easier* when it came time for them to decide how to create **well-balanced, fat-burning meals.**

OK, Should I ask WHY I'm Eating THIS?...

*Yes!!*

It's important to *know WHY you are eating or drinking specific nutrients*!

Especially if your *goal is a **flatter, tighter, more toned abdominal section.***

I say, if you don't know why you're eating and drinking a certain thing, <u>why do it</u>?

Like you, I've heard about a lot of **recommendations for foods and drinks to Make Weight-Loss Easier,** or **Give you a Flat Menopause Belly.**

Guess what!

*Instead, many of them keep a woman's belly fat, round, and non-flat.*

Here is my **5-QUESTION RULE.**

Before you eat or drink anything, *ask these, yourself!*:

## 5-Question Rule

◊ What is the Macronutrient Breakdown?

◊ Is this food or drink in line with my Flat Belly Goal?

◊ Is this product Processed or a Whole Food/Natural?

◊ Will this make my belly *Fatter* or *Flatter*?

◊ How many Calories are in this Drink or Food?

Once you have answers to **these 5 questions**, you will be very clear: *does the substance* **take you towards your flat belly or away.**

Now, I know: what you decide to do or eat, after answering these question, will be **impacted by your motivation *and* discipline.** That's what I covered in chapter 4.

BUT … beyond a shadow of a doubt, **<u>You'll Know</u>** the outcome or ramifications, should you decide to **consume OR reject the temptation** of any given food or drink on offer.

## How much to eat: Portion Control, Portion Control, Portion Control

I know that **you've heard about "portion control."**

Every magazine and fake online-nutritionist tells people that "the key to weigh loss is portion size."

Well, **I think that is <u>crap</u>!**

Everyone is different.

Each woman requires *a different quantity of calories* in order to support her healthy, active metabolism and hormonal balance.

I believe that **portion size should be correlated to a person's specific goals,** as well as to the **amount of calories** that she will consume throughout her day.

I always have my clients analyze their *RESTING METABOLIC RATE.*

From there, you, too, can *determine how many calories you require daily, in order to attain your goals*.

Here's a link where you can <u>calculate your RMR</u>. (It's at start-losing-weight-today.com/rmr.html.) You don't want to fall more than 200 calories below <u>your</u> personal RMR.

Here are some ***basic guidelines*** for selecting your own Menopause Success Triangle portion sizes.

~~~~~~~~

## Portion Size Guideline Based on 2000 Calories and 50/30/20 Macronutrient Ratio

1. CARBOHYDRATES: 50%
   - Starchy
   - Fibrous
   - Fruit / Simple Sugars

2. PROTEIN: 30%
   - Clean, Lean, Low Fat Protein Sources
   - White Meat, Fish, Bison, Turkey, Seafood
   - Whey & Casein Powder Mix

   (I discuss protein and other supplements in chapter 7; I often recommend protein shakes from Metaburn Nutrition, at metaburnnutrition.com.)

3. HEALTHY FATS: 20%
   - Oils
   - Nuts
   - Krill Oil
   - Fish Oils

~~~~~~

No matter which plan you develop for yourself, consider **shifting your personal eating habits so that you include** *more fresh foods* **across the day**, and eat *many small, regular meals* instead of just three larger ones.

Barbara and Lizz found that they could **transform their metabolism** and **reverse their weight gain** in part by making their lunches at home and bringing them to work, for example.

Lizz soon got other women to join her. She and her co-workers all had more energy and less body fat in just a few months!

~~~~~~~~~~~

As you begin to retool your nutrition plan, let me tell you how **certain foods can exacerbate or alleviate the top menopause symptoms.** Let's start with the ones that my clients mention the most.

*A. Insomnia*: **Tryptophan** is found in many foods. It is an amino acid that helps the brain to produce serotonin, which helps you to fall asleep. The ***Best Foods to address <u>insomnia</u> symptoms*** are:

*Turkey, soy, cod, egg whites, and omega-3 fatty acids* which can be found in *fish like salmon, trout and tuna.*

*Cherries.* They contain melatonin, a substance found in the body which helps to regulate sleep.

*Cottage cheese* contains tryptophan. If you don't consume dairy, you can also find tryptophan in *soy milk, tofu, hummus, and lentils.*

*Sesame seeds* are rich in tryptophan but high in carbohydrates. Sesame seeds do include a medium protein content, however, which makes them ***a perfect snack before bedtime.***

*Blueberries* can **help relieve stress**, and hence support restful sleep. They are loaded with vitamin C, which is a stress reducer.

*Almonds* also reduce stress with vitamins and minerals like vitamin B2, vitamin E, magnesium, and zinc.

**The Worst Foods** for anyone to consume who is suffering from menopause-related insomnia are:

*Caffeine*, which includes **coffee, tea, colas, and dark chocolate**—these all contain caffeine which may trigger hot flashes and affect your sleep. So, drink water instead, wherever possible. At very least, *avoid caffeine in the late afternoon and at night.*

*Alcohol* can increase hot flashes and affect sleep, mood, and weight. Limit yourself to *no more than one drink* a day. Preferably have alcohol in your diet only on special occasions.

*Large meals* can affect digestion, raise body temperature, and send signals to the brain that cause hot flashes. *Eating smaller meals* can help to reduce the number of hot flashes.

*B. Water Retention*: As I mentioned in chapter 1, water retention or bloating may be due to hormone fluctuations, the overproduction of estradiol, and the conversion of androgen (the "male" hormone) into estrogen through a process called *aromatization*, which increases with age and body weight.

According to Michelle Schoffro, PhD, clinical nutritionist, international best-selling author, and Doctor of Traditional Natural Medicine*, the Best Foods for bloating* are "dark leafy greens." They "help to deflate us after we've overindulged and put on a few pounds. They fuel your liver, which is your body's fat burning machine … No matter how many local, organic greens you're currently eating, consider eating more, because these guys are also loaded with antioxidants and fiber." Some other things to eat that counter water retention are: *Celery seeds; Parsley; Dandelion; Juniper berries; Asparagus; Artichokes; Melon;* and *Watercress*

Barbara found that she experienced much less bloating when she *increased her daily intake of water and herbal tea,* because they act as natural diuretics.

If you, too, suffer from water retention, **the Worst Foods** for you are *sugary and high-sodium foods.* **Frozen dinners** and **canned soups** have a shockingly high salt content, as do with processed foods and snack chips. All of these foods can cause water retention, swelling, and bloating.

The **sugar content** of many common foods may surprise you, even ones that we think of as healthy. I have my clients include the following items in their menopausal nutrition list only **with caution.**

*Breakfast Bars*: Some contain *as much as 13 grams of sugar in a single serving*. Just because they are organic doesn't mean that they can't contain nearly your entire daily quotient for sugar!

*Vitamin Water*: A bottle of vitamin water fuels your body with much more than just a dose of nutrients. That burst of energy that you feel when taking your last sip is just *a sugar high in disguise*. While these drinks can be a good choice soon after an intense workout, taking straight vitamins with a glass of water may be the better alternative.

*Bran Muffins*: There are **over 20 grams of sugar** in a bran muffin! Despite the fact that bran muffins to help you to reach your healthy fiber quota for the day, be sure not to mistake them for items that have a purely positive nutritional value.

*Dried Fruit:* Many of us want a quick snack, especially when we are on the go. Fruit is already naturally sweet; dried fruit concentrates that sugar into a higher sugar content for its portion size. *Choose a fresh piece of fruit instead of dried*, where possible; it is also easy to carry!

*Instant Oatmeal*: Although it's quick and easy, especially in the morning when you are in a hurry, the flavored variety of instant oatmeal can **contain 14**

**grams of sugar!** If you must do instant, hunt for the natural, low-sugar options.

*Flavored Yogurt*: While it might be a tasty, healthy boost for your metabolism, and even improve your immunity, certain commercial flavored yogurts also push you over the recommended daily sugar limit. A 6-ounce container of Yoplait Strawberry Yogurt, for example, is loaded with **27 grams of sugar.** Opt instead for plain yogurt, and add slices of fresh fruit for flavor.

Reducing or eliminating the amount of sugar and salt that you consume from food and beverages will help you to decrease bloating, and keep your sugar levels from rising into sugar highs, then plummeting rapidly in ways that cause mood swings.

*C. Mood Swings/Hot Flashes:* Clean, healthy foods can make marked changes in your moods, and free you from the ups and downs that accompany high fat/high sugar diets.

For example, **when you feel sad, it can be due to something that you need** in your diet. Magnesium is a mineral that's known for producing serotonin. Good sources of magnesium include: *halibut; almonds, cashews, and unprocessed peanut butter; spinach; black eyed peas, lentils, kidney and pinto beans; baked potatoes,* and *long grain brown rice. Bananas* also aid the brain in its release of serotonin.

When you have a menopausal **tendency to feel angry,** *avoid* certain foods like **spicy peppers and hot high-flavor spices.** This choice can reduce not only those fired-up feelings, but hot flashes, too. If your body is already heated, you don't need anything else to help "fuel the flame."

When my clients AnnaMaria and Michelle complained about **lacking clarity**, they increased the amount of *blueberries, strawberries, and açaí berries* in their diet. These fruits **activate the brain's natural "housekeeping"** mechanism. Super fruits clean up and

**recycle toxic proteins** that are **linked to memory loss and brain fog**, along with other over-emotional reactions.

Utah State University researchers say that those women who follow the following diet score the highest on memory, attention-span, and problem-solving skills:

*Whole grains*—at least **_three whole-grain_ foods per day**

*Low-fat or fat-free dairy products*

*Nuts, seeds, and dry beans*

*Vegetables and fruit*—at least **eight servings per day**. (Only 11% of Americans consume even the USDA minimum of five fruits and vegetables daily, says a 2007 report.)

*Fish and poultry; minimal lean red meat*

*Limited fats and sweets*

~~~~~~~~~~

The bottom line about looking seriously at your diet and nutrition as you build a successful menopause lifestyle is that **you are what you eat**! Check out the Menopause Diet, too, in chapter 6.

## 2. EXERCISE

When Denise began to work with me, she was 52 years old, and not all that concerned about losing weight. What she wanted was *to feel healthy, fit, and active again.*

What my menopausal exercise plan did for Denise, along with my coaching and support, was motivate her to stick to a program, and consistently build her strength. She became progressively stronger and more agile.

The *change was RADICAL!*

When she started to work with me, she **couldn't do <u>any</u> push-ups** at all, and was **only working out once each week**.

After following this MENOPAUSE SUCCESS TRIANGLE WORKOUT PLAN, she is *up to* _ten_ *push-ups* easily, and also squeezes in my recommended _**3-4**_ _**thirty-minute workouts**_ *every week.*

Jillian, Barbara, and Deborah embraced my MENOPAUSE SUCCESS TRIANGLE WORKOUT PLAN because they were concerned about *a general increase in their body fat,* and, specifically, in changes to their amount of _**abdominal fat**_.

Here's what all the studies show:

> *Being more active is directly linked to losing or keeping off weight during menopause.*

A National Institute of Health report found that people who participated in aerobic activities every day for **10 or more minutes** had *six fewer inches around their waistlines,* compared to people who did no exercise.

I found the same thing to be true, and its effects rippled out into each woman's full menopause experience! For example, as my three clients **added to** or **increased their level of exercise,** they noticed *dramatic reductions in their symptoms of menopause,* particularly their hot flashes and insomnia.

I believe in the Golden Rule of Exercise: no matter what you do, how you feel, or how packed your schedule, *you deserve to give your body an hour of your time each day in order to keep it in good shape*.

Exercise enhances mood. Denise and Susanne noticed that they *experienced __many__ more disturbances to their mood and sleep*, plus more menopause-related brain fog **when they <u>didn't have enough activity</u>** in their daily routines.

These are called *vasomotor symptoms*. They are *MUCH less common among menopausal women who are physically active*. Regular exercise improves cognitive function, enhances mood, **and** promotes daytime alertness.

## *DON'T COMPROMISE!*

The Workout Plan that I am going to share with you has:

- ▶ Regulated Jillian's metabolism
- ▶ Increased Barbara's blood circulation
- ▶ Reduced Deborah's hot flashes

It will help you to **feel refreshed**, plus **lower your risk of heart attack and stroke** by keeping your level of blood cholesterol low.

In women over the age of 45, being inactive leads to an *increase in the level of "bad" cholesterol* and a decrease in "good" cholesterol. It *increases blood pressure,* and leads to an *increased risk* of a wide range of diseases.

Women in their 40s and 50s become more susceptible to **metabolic syndrome, heart attack**, and other **cardiovascular disease.**

SO ... if you don't already have a program for moving and stretching, it is **critical that you consider adopting the** WORKOUT PLAN **that I propose below.**

You'll also find that your joints and muscles are stronger, and that your depression and anxiety are lessened as you increase your activity level. Over time, this program will lower your risk of osteoporosis, improve insulin resistance, and, of course, help you to lose and maintain your weight, during and after menopause.

### 5 Components of the Menopause Success Triangle Workout Plan

There are *five components* to this WORKOUT PLAN. It covers *21 Days.*

When I first met Barbara, she was 56 years old, post-menopausal, and *very* **busy** as a mom and community activist. Her challenge was that *she had not been working out at all,* and found that she had *gained 25-30 pounds* in just the prior two years, alone.

I helped her to analyze her nutrition plan, but she was a former Weight Watcher's rep, so she knew how to recognize her macronutrient needs, and how to reincorporate smart, healthy eating into her lifestyle.

The **key to her reducing the unhealthy fat** that was in her diet was for her to **cook at home more**; this reduced the number of times that she and her husband ate out each week. I also had her commit to **eating a good breakfast every morning**, one that included more **protein to kick-start her metabolism** for the day.

Then, we began to follow this 21-DAY WORKOUT PLAN, *in rotation, 3-4 times each week*.

Barbara managed to set aside at least **30 minutes for every work-out session.**

**<u>She lost 22 pounds during our first 14 weeks!</u>**

There are **five basic components** to every fitness plan that I design for menopausal women. These elements are **combined in different proportions**. They **incorporate different activities** to stay effective and interesting.

**Ideally,** a menopausal woman who wants to achieve realistic, healthy results will **dedicate at least 30-40 minutes to these exercises at least 3-4 times each week**.

**GOOD NEWS!** <u>**30-minute workouts are just great for the super busy woman with time constraints**</u>.

On days when you have more time, though, you can easily increase your cardio or another one of these five plan components:

*A. Metabolic resistance*: these are **aerobic exercises combined with strength training**.

An example would be the **dumbbell squats** that I have Barbara do, along with **overhead presses,** for a specified amount of time. Exercises in this category *increase her heart rate above normal,* which in turn *stimulate her body's fat-burning ability*. They also trigger her **POC, or Pulse Oxygen Consumption,** which helps her body to *continue* *burning fat for 24-48 hours after each one of her 30-minute workouts*.

*B. Strength Training*: the objective of these exercises is to *do multiple sets for a specified number of reps,* in order to *increase lean muscle and maintain bone mass.*

This was a critical component of the program that I designed for both Barbara and Denise. Here is an important fact for you to remember: **<u>menopausal women need to work with heavier weights (above 5 pounds) in order to activate their metabolism.</u>**

Denise found that the strength-building exercises in the initial 21-Day Workout Plan, including the use of **weight machines, dumbbells, exercise bands**, and **yoga,** motivated her to stick with the strength progression that I prescribed, so that she got the most out of her time and training.

\*\**My #1 secret for helping women over age 45* expand their activity to improve their metabolism and weight loss *is to increase their weights*.\*\*

I have my clients do *8-20 reps for 4-5 sets, with 15-45-second rest periods* in between.

Barbara and Denise got great results by **including weight-resistance training in their workouts at least two or three times each week.**

*C. Cardio training*: Lizz and Michelle were both very familiar with the ***heart-healthy benefits of including cardio*** exercise in their workout routines. Cardio **increases respiratory rates, and stimulates both aerobic and cardiovascular strength.**

But, my clients ***weren't yet sure which cardio activities were best*** for them, or ***how much to do***.

I encouraged them to **add 30 minutes of cardio** exercise to their routines **at least three days each week.**

Michelle was a walker. You can walk anytime, most anywhere. In the warm months, she would also play tennis.

Lizz liked to **alternate her cardio** between a variety of low- and medium-impact options like **swimming, cycling**, and **aerobics.**

Nadi was a 44-year-old client who had never worked out before she started to train with me. She **increased her lean muscle and decreased her body fat 5%** by **starting dance classes** and **yoga** as her cardio activities, in partnership with **adding new strength training and metabolic resistance exercises** to her workouts.

I wanted Lizz and Denise to **blend the two important types of cardio training**. When you create your own 21-Day Workout Plan, be sure to include a mix of both of these cardio types:

*Interval training or burst training:* Lizz did **20-second "bursts" of all-out sprints** on the elliptical trainer. Or she **pedaled intensely for 20 seconds** on the stationary bike, followed by 10 seconds of recovery. On her burst-training days, I had her repeat this sequence for **8-12 rounds**. By then, she had met her total cardio needs for the day!

*Steady-state cardio* is ***20-30 minutes of any cardio activity that is maintained at a steady pace*** on the **treadmill, elliptical trainer**, or **walking/running** outside. Just be sure that you are working hard enough. I asked Denise to make sure that she could ***pass the "cell-phone test"*** when she did her steady-state cardio: she had to push herself hard enough so that she couldn't workout ***and*** maintain a regular conversation through her heavy breathing. If you can have a full-on conversation during your cardio sessions, then you aren't walking fast enough!

**D.** *Mobility and flexibility* are critical components of the Menopause Success Triangle Workout Plan. With Denise, Lizz, and Jillian, I always began our workout sessions with exercises that ***moved their body through a full range of motion for each joint.***

**Dynamic mobility exercises** include arm swings, knee pulls, overhead reaches, side lunges, and step-back lunges. The key for me is that you ***stretch and expand your muscles*** while you stimulate your lymphatic drainage system, which flushes out body toxins.

Each workout with these women ended with **flexibility stretches,** which are **static, extended 20-second stretches of each muscle group.** Then, ***you go a little deeper*** until you reach your maximum stretch.

I always include these stretches as **part of the cool-down process**, because, until that point in a workout, I want each client to activate and contract their muscles, not yet relax and stretch them.

*E. Rest and Recovery*: When I talked to Denise about including this **one new thing into her routine**, she wasn't sure if it was necessary. But it was!

In a big way, I attribute **regular massages** to her newfound sense of health and well-being.

I am a true believer in **scheduling regular massages** during menopause, primarily because they keep your tissues and muscles loose and relaxed.

In addition, I had Nadi and Lizz each buy **a foam roller to use at home,** too. They use them to do self-myofascial release. This **smooths out any adhesions that you pick up in your ligaments, or in the tendons of your legs and upper back**.

Nadi has her roller in her bedroom, and uses it on her legs, hips, and lower back.

Lizz had **upper back syndrome** from working at a desk over a computer., She alleviated a lot of neck pain and rounded shoulders by rolling slowly and gently but consistently over her adhesions, knots, and tight spots, re-oxygenating her muscles, and allowing them to move freely in the fascia that sheath her tendons and other connective tissue.

## How to Create YOUR WORKOUT PLAN

First, let me give you the 21-day Menopause Success Triangle Workout Calendar.

Sometimes, starting with a <u>picture</u> can help you to make sense of things! So, here you go:

| Sunday | Monday | Tuesday | Wedneday | Thursday | Friday | Saturday |
|---|---|---|---|---|---|---|
| Optional Cardio : Stretch : Prep for the Week | A | Rest | B | Rest | A | Cardio A |
| Optional Cardio : Stretch : Prep for the Week | Cardio B | B | Rest | A | Cardio A | B |
| Optional Cardio : Stretch : Prep for the Week | A | Cardio B | B | Rest | A | Cardio A |
| | | | | | | |
| NOTE: You can repeat this same program for upto 6-8 Weeks and continue to receive gains. After that You body will have adapted to the work and no long give you the same bang for your buck... | | | | | | |

You can also **Print This Chart Out** at this website: www.MenopauseSuccessTriangle.com.

Don't worry: I'm going to **make this totally clear in the following section!**

My 21-Day Workout Plan **spans 3 weeks, and then it is repeated … Forever!**

**Each time that you begin your 21-day Workout Plan over again, you have the opportunity to shuffle around the exercises, to extend the number of reps, or to up your weight levels**.

The idea here is to *build a solid weekly work-out plan* that challenges and inspires you, and that helps you to attain your fitness and fat-loss goals.

There are **two basic strength and conditioning workouts:**

- ▶ Workout A
- ▶ Workout B

There are **two to four different versions of Cardio training,** which I discuss more below

For this calendar I call them:

▶ Cardio A
▶ Cardio B

REST days are *super important*.

I **mix in rest days** between workouts, because a lot of the *important work happens in your body on those days.*

On rest days, you **recover** and go through the **adaptation process**, which I consider the real work for your body. In those hours between workouts, *you heal, and your system has a chance to adjust your hormones*. REST also *gets you into a healthy state,* so that you are ready to go again on your next scheduled training day.

SUNDAYS are *always left unscheduled* in my training plan, but you have a few options there:

▶ One option for Sunday is to **do any sort of additional cardio workout, like a hike or bike ride.**
▶ Another is to **dedicate Sunday to a stretching routine**, or maybe to do a **yoga** or **pilates** class

that balances the strength- and core-conditioning that you do on other workout days.

▶ The third idea is to **make it a pure rest day**: recuperate, maybe **schedule a massage**, and then prepare for the week ahead.

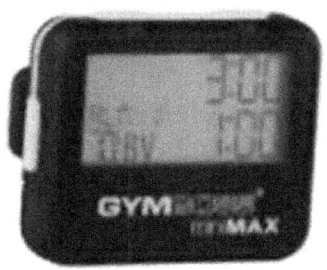

**What kind of equipment do you need?**

Not much!

Stuff that you would find at any gym. But these items are also very easy to stock, yourself, at home:

- 5-, 8-, and 12-pound dumbbells
- A jump rope
- 8-pound medicine ball
- An alarm, stopwatch, or timer; it can be on your phone, or check out Gymboss.com: they have a great little Gymboss Interval Timer that is super useful
- Water bottle

- Sweat towel
- Yoga mat for cool down and stretching

That's it!

**I want to say something again: *RAISE THE LEVEL OF THE WEIGHTS THAT YOU WORK OUT WITH.***

WHY?!

In menopause, you certainly **don't need to worry about bulking up**—your hormones don't support that; nobody's body does naturally, really. But **you do want to have** toned arms, burn more fat, and **balance your hormones** naturally.

To do that, <u>you need to lift heavier weights</u>, ones that really challenge you.

I'll tell you when to do your weight lifting, below, during the descriptions of my workout plans.

But, **whenever you're called to pick up a weight for an exercise,** be sure that you can still **<u>feel some real resistance</u>**. If you don't, **move on up** to the next level!

## HERE'S THE CALENDAR

### WEEK 1:

- Day 1, begin with Workout A (I outline it below)
- Then take a rest day, Day 2
- Day 3, do Workout B.
- Rest on Day 4
- Repeat Workout A on Day 5
- Finish your week on Day 6 with your Cardio A workout (also described below!)
- SUNDAY ... TAKE OFF!

### WEEK 2:

- Start Day 1 with your Cardio B workout
- On Day 2, repeat your Workout B
- Rest on Day 3
- Day 4, return to Workout A
- Day 5, do Cardio A
- Finish the week with a second round of Workout B
- SUNDAY ... OFF

### WEEK 3:

- Day 1 begin with Workout A
- Do Cardio B on Day 2
- Workout B on Day 3

- Rest on Day 4
- Day 5, repeat Workout A
- Finish the week with Cardio A on Day 6
- SUNDAY ... OFF

Here's how that looks, in 21 days. Then read on to see what you do for each of these Workouts!

Day 1: Workout A

Day 2: Rest

Day 3: Workout B

Day 4: Rest

Day 5: Workout A

Day 6: Cardio A

Day 7: Fun Sunday – yoga, Cardio C, stretch

Day 8: Cardio B

Day 9: Workout B

Day 10: Rest

Day 11: Workout A

Day 12: Cardio A

Day 13: Workout B

Day 14: Fun Sunday — Yoga, Rest, Cardio, Stretch

Day 15: Workout A

Day 16: Cardio B

Day 17: Workout B

Day 18: Rest

Day 19: Workout A

Day 20: Cardio A

Day 21: Fun Sunday — Yoga, Cardio, Rest

Start OVER!

## What are these "Workouts" and "Cardios A&B"!?

### WORKOUT A:

► **Warm Up – 5-8 minutes:** Get your joints and muscles ready to do work with a simple series of *Dynamic mobility exercises* that move your body at a controlled pace through a full range of motion for each joint. Remember: these exercises can include arm swings, knee pulls, overhead reaches, side lunges, moving in dynamic stretches, and step-back lunges, that warm and expand your muscles while flushing the body of toxins through your lymphatic drainage system.

**Here is a great video sample Dynamic Warm-up by my friend Uri Elkaim, on YouTube.

(*For paperback readers, you can find the video online right here:* http://www.youtube.com/watch?v=hkRtMVzRDCc&feature= player_detailpage)

Yuri gives you some excellent warm-up ideas; the video will help you to visualize the process. *It's very important to start every workout this way!*

So—spend 5-8 minutes swinging your arms in circles in both directions. Lift your knee really high and pull it up as you stand on one leg, then alternate to the other. Do jumping jacks. Also, lunges forward and back are great dynamic warm-up movements, as well.

**This isn't ballistic:** it's *not about how fast you do these warm-ups, nor about the number of reps*, like in other parts of your work-out.

And **don't hold any movement very long** as you move forward, backwards, and through the transverse planes. Your goal is just to *get your body parts working fluidly* and effortlessly, as you gradually increase your core body temperature. Together, these goals and movements will protect your muscles from injury.

▶ **SCP 1: Your First Strength Conditioning Phase.**

This is *a circuit of 4 exercises*, each one done for *30 seconds.* You are going to *do 2 rounds of these four SCP exercises,* with a *30-second rest* between each round.

Like every exercise in the CP and Core portions of my workouts, **determine your own intensity**, and modify it to match, and then challenge, your personal fitness level.

A. **Front Straight-leg Kicks:** Stand up tall and straight, with a nice neutral spine, and lift your leg straight up, alternating left and right.

**B. Jumping Jacks or Marching in Place.**

**C. Squats:** These are so great for the three major muscle groups in your legs—the quads on the front of your thigh, the hammies on the back, and the glutes in your butt. Do 30 seconds of squats, like you're sitting back in a chair, knees never extending out past your toes.

**D. Push-ups:** Go for 30 seconds, preferably on your toes, but on your knees with a tight straight core if you need that assistance. Blend wide-elbow push-ups with the yoga variety, where you keep your elbows tight against your rib cage (tougher! But great for your arm definition!) Squat—great for quads (front of thighs), hams (back of thighs), and glutes (butt)—30 seconds

**E. Rest:** Only 30 seconds!

**F. Then, Repeat A - E.**

▶ **SCP 2: Your *Second* Strength Conditioning Phase**

This is another circuit of 4 exercises. It alternates between working your upper body, then your lower body, in order to include a peripheral heart-training system. As one body part rests, the other is called into action, then we switch. Do each exercise below for 30 seconds.

A. **Wall stick-ups:** These create mobility in your shoulders so that you can cut through common tension in your neck and cervical spine area. Stand straight up against a wall, and put your arms straight up, like you're in a bank "stick up."

Now, lower them all the way down the wall, depressing your arms straight to your thighs, but keeping your wrist, elbow and back glued as close to the wall as possible. Then lift them back up to the top, and back down again.

If you feel true stiffness or pain, here or in any exercise, **stop**. If you're just a little sore (or you feel it the next day, as Delayed Onset Muscle Soreness), that is OK.

But the idea is *never to push you to pain*. You may only start out doing 5-10 stick-ups, for example, and then ease up to the full 30 seconds, twice, over your first 21 days. But your body *will adapt* to the new stress and strength demands that we are making on it!

**B. Dumbbell Alternate Front Lunges:** OK, first, you need weights for this exercise.

*Remember what I said about your dumbbells?* Use at least 8#, but progress to 10-12-15# as soon as possible. You'll burn more fat, and you will naturally increase your hormones that much more quickly, by raising your weight level.

Now, hold one weight in each hand by your side, dangling like heavy suitcases. Step <u>forward</u> with your left leg and drop down with it into a lunge, lowering yourself with control and again keeping the left knee behind your toe, with the right leg straight behind you.

Then, push through your left heel to stand straight back up, legs together. Now, step forward with the opposite/right leg, and repeat. Continue on the left, then the right leg, for 30 seconds.

**C. Rest, then Wall Stick-ups:** Rest for 30 seconds, and then do a 2nd set of stick-ups.

**D. Dumbbell Front Lunges:** Do a 2$^{nd}$ set of alternating lunges for 30 seconds.

**E. Chair Dip:** This is for your triceps, and firms up the back of your arms beautifully. It really keeps those "bat wings" away! Begin by putting resistance on your triceps muscles. You can use any chair seat in your home, for example, or a bench in the park or at the gym. Just put your hands on the seat beside you, hover your back in front of the seat, and dip down and up for 30 seconds. Keep your back straight and close to the chair as it goes up and down.

▶ Core Phase:

There are two exercises in each Workout's Core Phase. The first has two sides—hold each side for 30 seconds, then do the second exercise for 30 seconds.

**A. Side Plank Hold**. Lie on your left side with either your right hand or forearm on the ground. Lift your hips, legs straight, and hold for 30 seconds.

Then roll over and repeat on the right for 30 seconds. If your arms or back feel too much strain at first, you can modify this by doing it on the side of your knees, instead of balancing on the edges of your feet; this will shorten the lever, and the burden on your arm.

But be sure that the line from your leg to your neck is a straight, taut one; you will work your side muscles, the obliques.

B. **Russian Twist:.** Sit on floor with your knees in soft bend. Hold your medicine ball, a 10-pound dumbbell, or a heavy bag of flour. Lean back slightly into a c-curve, then rotate right to left and the back for 30 seconds, holding your abs in that slight tuck.

▶ The Finisher: After every Core Phase, and before the wonderful cool-down stretch, comes your *finisher.*

This phase of your workout is designed to metabolically burn fat, and to push you into what we call the "Afterburn Effect," where this high-intensity metabolism continues for 48-72 hours post-workout, and your body continues to burn fat as though you were still exercising.

Great, right?

But the only way to kick-start that Effect is to do this final push, following on the overload principle where you work out at maximum capacity for a short duration.

***Here is your Workout A Finisher:*** *Hit these!* No Relaxed Pace yet! Bang these out as fast as you can, with proper form, and then *jump* to the next one.

A. **8 Push-ups**
B. **8 Squats**
C. **8 Sit-ups**
D. **8 Medicine ball chops Right,** where you swing your ball or an 8-10 # dumbbell from low from alongside of your right knee diagonally across your body to your left shoulder and back. These work your internal and external oblique muscles, further strengthening your core.
E. **8 Medicine ball chops, Left.**

▶ **Cool Down Stretch:**
Finish Workout A with 5 minutes of relaxed breathing in order to lower the cortisone level in your body, and cool everything down. Include static stretches, like I described above. Unlike

your dynamic warm-up, these motions are held for 15-30 seconds first, then take your stretch a little deeper before you move on to stretch another side, or part, of your body.

## WORKOUT B:

▶ **Warm Up—5-8 minutes:** Get your joints and muscles ready to do work with a series of *Dynamic mobility exercises* that move your body through a full range of motion for each joint. Check our Uri's Elkaim's video link on YouTube (see above) if you want some more great ideas.

▶ **Strength/Conditioning Phase:**
Here is the series of exercises for your SCP in Workout B:

A. **Side Lunges:** For 30 seconds, lunge to your right and then to your left, alternating. Continue to check your alignment so that your butt stays back, and your knees remain behind your toes.

B. **Jump-rope or Running in Place:** 30 seconds. Pick your poison. And *push*—you should be breathing hard throughout this SC Phase. Like always, pace yourself. Stop if you feel dizzy or nauseous, and adjust your pace. But for maximum healthy effect, don't hold back.

C. **Lying Hip Bridges:** Like the Side Plank in Workout A, but lower your hips to the matt, and then raise them to plank on each side for 30 seconds. Then, switch sides.

D. **Anterior Dumbbell Press:** Do these floor presses with 10-12# weights.

E. **Split Squat:** Your left leg is forward, your right leg back. Hold a dumbbell in each hand like a suitcase as you lower into a lunge, then, as you push yourself up, do a bicep curl before lowering arms and knee back down again. Repeat for 30 seconds, and then switch to your second side.

F. **Dumbbell Deadlift Lateral Raise:** Choose lighter weights for this—maybe 5-8#. This exercise is hip-dominant for your glutes and hamstrings so, standing straight, lower both weights down below your kneecaps.

Keeping your back very straight, stand up straight as you lift your arms out to the side, eyes out in front, pushing through your heels. Then, lower the arms again and repeat for 30 seconds.

**G. Dumbbell kickbacks:** This is another exercise to build your arm strength for wearing those tank tops and strapless dresses. Using those same lighter weights, lean forward slightly and bend your elbows into right angles alongside your ribs like wings. Straighten them backwards behind you, using your triceps, then bend for 30 seconds. These will make your arms look *fabulous:* strong, but not bulky.

**H. Dumbbell side bends:** To complete your Workout B arm conditioning, take your left arm and put your hand behind your head. Put a dumbbell in your right hand. Lower that dumbbell to the right, with your elbow pointing to the ceiling, then come back down, pointing the elbow to the floor.

You are only working one arm at a time—that is so important for your lateral spinal flexion. Bending your elbow, lower the weight to the right until your left elbow points to the ceiling, then lower your elbow until it points to the floor. Do this for 30 seconds on the left, then 30 seconds on the right.

▶ CORE: OK, here are your two core exercises for Workout B.

**A. Reverse Slow Crunch:** These are *great* for the lower part of your abs, below the belly button—an area that many women consider problematic. I love having you do *lots* of these! Lie on your back with your hands and feet flat on the floor, your knees pressed tightly together. Slowly draw your knees up towards your shoulders, lifting your hips just slightly off of the ground, and then lower them back to the floor with control. Repeat this for 30 seconds.

**B. Dynamic Plank.** This is very cool. We all know what a plank is, where you balance on your elbows, legs straight behind you with your back straight and your belly button pulled tight into your spine. Make it *dynamic*! Rotate your pelvis to the right, then the left, and then back again for 30 seconds as you maintain a neutral spine. This taxes your core to the fullest as you work internal and external obliques. An ideal exercise for slimming your waist.

▶ **FINISHER.** Here is your Workout B Finisher series:

**A. 8 Dumbbell Y Presses:** Hold your dumbbells near your shoulders, one in each hand, and press them out overhead and up diagonally in a V.

**B. 8 squats**

**C. 8 Medicine Ball Chops, Left**

**D. 8 Medicine Ball Chops, Right**

▶ **REST:** Cool down with at least 5 minutes of relaxing, stretching, and deep breathing.

## CARDIO A:

A brisk 30-minute walk

## CARDIO B:

30 minutes on the stationary bike

## CARDIO C:

Jazz or hip-hop dance class

## CARDIO D:

Swim or Row for 30 minutes

CARDIO E:

30 minutes on the elliptical machine, or treadmill

The ***goal of your Cardio Workouts*** is to get your **body moving and heart rate up** using whatever equipment you have at your disposal. ***Do whatever activity you enjoy.***

**PUT A NUMBER** of <u>**different cardio workouts**</u> into rotation, so that you never tire of doing them when your Cardio Day appears in the 21-Day Menopause Success Triangle Workout Plan. Mix, match, and define your own!

~~~~~~~

One last thing that you might want to consider as you build and bolster your menopausal exercise routine this:

***Should you work out with a trainer or coach***?

Denise needed someone to motivate her to do the *strength progressions* that built up the full-body fitness that she needed.

Lizzette found that her menopause coach pushed her to work harder, and helped her to *set, and then achieve, her fitness and nutrition goals*.

A **PERSONAL MENOPAUSE COACH** is **a fitness trainer who has extensive knowledge about women's health** and who **specializes in exercise for menopausal women**.

This type of trainer can *guide you through a healthier and more comfortable menopause transition* by developing your workouts *based on your individual* lab work, health history, *and* lifestyle.

They establish an exercise routine for you that is *tailored specifically to suit your needs*, since no two women are exactly alike when it comes to signs and symptoms of menopause.

The best coaches also *coordinate their efforts with your health-care provider*, and *assist in injury prevention, motivation, strength building*, and *safe weight-loss monitoring*.

~~~~~~~

Physical activity is a critical part of the Menopause Success Triangle. Unlike dieting, which only affects the amount of calories that you take in, physical activity *helps your body to burn more calories,* not only while you're working out, but **afterwards, as well**.

As you build more muscle, you will also **increase your metabolism.** The faster your menopause metabolism, as I discussed in chapter 3, the more calories that you will burn per hour. The more calories that you burn per hour, the more weight you can lose (or at least, not gain).

The combination of exercise and proper nutrition can dramatically reduce the symptoms of menopause, plus improve your emotional state and help you to better cope with stress. Like Lizz, Barbara, and Denise, you will find that you have increased energy, and more pleasant, productive days.

## 3. STRESS REDUCTION

The third component of my approach to a successful menopause experience is <u>**just as important as the other two**</u>.

When Jillian came to work with me, **she was stressed**.

Her work and family obligations were very time-consuming, and she was experiencing severe menopausal symptoms, like **brain fog** and **edginess**. We did a nutritional analysis together and adjusted her diet, then I added some regular strength-training and metabolic resistance to her workout regime. But I was also very keen *to lower her stress levels dramatically.*

I shared with Jillian some critical information about the **causes and consequences of stress during**

**menopause**, both on the physiological and psychological levels.

Then I introduced Jillian to *yoga and meditation.* I believe that these are the **best "medicine" for alleviating stress,** and for fighting the sorts of menopausal symptoms that bothered her the most.

***Stress is a state of mind that believes that everything is an emergency.***

Stress doesn't have to produce anxiety or even be perceived consciously for your internal organs to believe that there is an **emergency situation**.

Of course, there is "good" stress and "bad" stress.

Unfortunately, ***our body doesn't distinguish between the two.*** It reacts the same way, whether stress is physical, chemical, or emotional.

Our bodies were built to respond to stress. But as it becomes chronic, ***the stress-regulating parts of the body begin to fatigue.*** Then, they **no longer work as well** as intended. Oprah has a great online stress test (there's a link to it in my resources chapter, too). It can help you *analyze your own lifestyle stress levels.* **Check it out at oprah.com/spirit/the-stress-detector-test**.

Jillian already knew that **stress didn't *feel* right**. She described it as an emotional state of feeling **tight, pressured, edgy, over her head**, and **out of sorts**.

Can you relate to that?

It probably won't surprise you to learn, as she did, that stress has *an actual physical effect on our body and its ability to heal* and remain youthful.

Stress **frays our telomeres**, which are the ends of our DNA strands that protect our genetic data. Healthy telomeres ensure that our chromosomes divide correctly, and that they don't lose small pieces of critical genetic material that tell our tissues how to repair themselves and ward off disease. *Healthy telomeres are crucial to the DNA replication process*.

When they **fray or shorten through stress**, however, our DNA does not duplicate completely, and <u>**we see signs of aging or illness.**</u>

The great news that I shared with Jillian is this: **telomeres can be repaired,** like other parts of our bodies. Stress reduction and physical activity were the first steps to her rejuvenation, and will be to yours, too.

Stress (whether emotional, chemical, or physical) is **processed in a part of the brain called the** *hypothalamus*.

The hypothalamus sends a message to the anterior *pituitary gland,* which is a small gland in the brain that helps to regulate all of your hormones. As the pituitary gland secretes hormones into the blood that signal stress, **another gland called the** *adrenal gland* **responds by secreting cortisol.**

*Cortisol* is designed to **control the body's response to stress by stimulating the body to calm down.**

Jillian and Lizzette experienced symptoms when they produced ***too much cortisol*** over a long period of time. As a result, they had **disrupted sleep, poor digestion, weight gain, poor memory**, and more.

Excess cortisol **can also remove the hormone *progesterone*** from your body. You are **already experiencing depletion** or fluctuations through the menopause process.

When Nadi and Lisa discovered stress-related progesterone imbalances in their blood tests, they ***connected it to some of their* weight gain,** to the memory problems that we call **"brain fog,"** and to **fatigue.**

Part of what I did with Jillian and Nadi was to *reduce their stress through* diet modification, nutritional supplementation, *and* exercise.

This helped to ***re-balance their cortisol, estrogen, and progesterone.***

I also discovered that Lizzette, along with my client Michelle, was *suffering from adrenal fatigue*. I addressed their stress in part by **explaining the relationship between their *adrenal glands* and their menopausal symptoms**.

The **adrenal glands** are two small glands, each about the size of a large grape, situated on top of the kidneys. Their main *purpose is to help the body cope with stress* and survive.

As certain hormones produced by the adrenal glands diminish, the *body is no longer able to deal with stress* the same way.

*Aldosterone* is an important hormone that can be controlled through stress reduction. That will *reduce adrenal fatigue,* according to Dr. Lam of the Adrenal Fatigue Center.

When stress increases aldosterone, it *interferes with sodium and potassium levels, causing the* water

**retention, lethargy, *and* inability to lose weight** that Lizzette and Michelle described to me.

I had both of these women **introduce yoga** into their fitness routines. Their new yoga practice went a long way towards addressing their ***adrenal fatigue syndrome***.

~~~~~~~~~~~~~~~~~~~~~~~~~

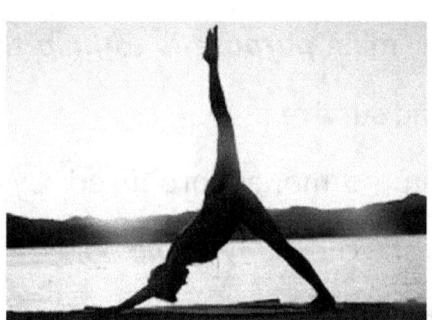

*YOGA* has long been established as an extremely effective way to reduce stress. It also increases strength and over-all body health.

Yoga can have a ***hugely positive impact on your youthfulness and fitness*** specifically during menopause.

Because you are losing the hormone estrogen which keeps skin taut and young, a practice like yoga *facilitates better blood circulation;* this in turn helps the body to *stay younger longer*.

Increased blood circulation not only ensures that your skin remains more firm, but it also *prevents cellulite deposits along the arteries,* thereby reducing the risk of heart attack.

**Yoga means "union":** the union of mind, body, and spirit. It involves *moving the body in ways that help you to feel peaceful and connected* with everything around you.

It is an exercise **comprised of postures, or *asanas***, that are practiced together in 60- or 90-minute sessions.

Jillian described **feeling more open and alive** once she took up yoga. It certainly can *rebalance your perspective, improve your physiology, build strength*, and *open you to experience all aspects of your menopause in harmony*.

For any woman like Nadi or Michelle who is middle-aged or beyond, yoga can be a form of **menopause medicine.**

Yoga helped Michelle to ***adjust to the various hormonal changes*** that were taking place in her body, because it *balances the endocrine system*, so it **reduced** the effects of her **night sweats and mood swings.**

Nadi found that yoga *gave her a peaceful energy* that **alleviated some of her fatigue.**

Yoga can be a wonderful, challenging workout, as well as a relaxing, de-stressing one. It actually **makes you *stronger* and *more flexible*** at the same time, by **building your core strength, challenging your upper body power,** and **stretching joints and muscles** that need to **avoid age-related stiffness.**

A regular practice of yoga poses—sitting, standing, lying down, forward bends, backbends, and twists—*activates and stimulates all of the organs, glands,*

**cells, and tissues in your body**. Thus, through yoga, you will not only keep your weight in check: you will also help to **keep your body healthy, fit, and stress-free**.

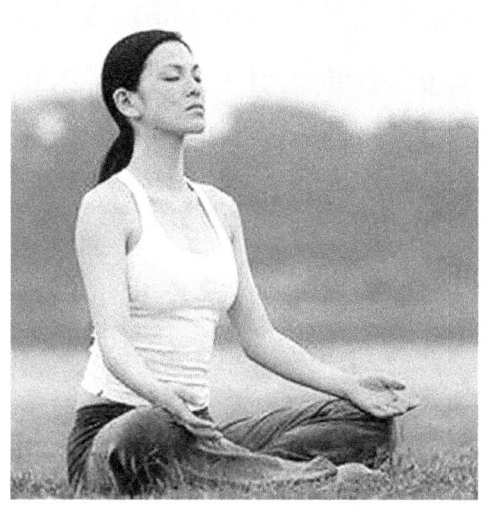

**Meditation** is the other key activity that I introduced to Michelle and many other women. It, too, works to **lower the emotional stress that accompanyies menopause**.

Scientists believe that meditation **switches the body from active (sympathetic nervous system) mode to restful (parasympathetic nervous system) mode,** which dilates blood vessels and improves blood flow in the body.

There are numerous forms of meditation that you can choose, but I encourage my clients **to take twenty minutes each morning or evening, at minimum**, and **experience the calming of the mind** that comes with meditation.

*The process involves "letting go" of yourself and your surroundings, projecting yourself positively, and allowing stressful moments to pass.*

Michelle enjoyed focusing on a simple *combination of breathing exercises and positive affirmations* from chapter 4, as her meditation practice.

Jillian responded really well to a more active mind-meditation, where she *visualized positive healing in various parts of her body* that had become uncomfortable or that were changing. She always ended her sessions *by focusing deep breathing on her heart center or "heart chakra,"* and found that the results very relaxing, overall.

I love the way that meditation reduces cardiovascular risks in my clients who are experiencing high blood pressure or other physical stressors during menopause. Because meditation relaxes the mind and body, it releases strain on the heart that accompanies stress; in many cases, it also lowers blood pressure.

As Jillian and Michelle's stress levels came down through their practice of meditation, they *developed a naturally healthier outlook on life.*

Studies have shown that **meditation also boosts your body's level of** *melatonin,* a hormone that *increases immunity to illness,* and that can *improve sleep quality, too*. Jillian definitely reported feeling more refreshed and also sleeping more deeply, once she began her yoga and meditation.

My Menopause Success Triangle Plan for Lizz, Deborah, Barbara and Michelle *addressed de-stressing just as much as it did nutrition and exercise*

*WHY?*

Because I believe *__that strongly__* that STRESS has a serious impact on your menopausal symptoms and healthy lifestyle.

I want each of my clients to *enjoy the wonders of life and the beauties of the world without stress and fatigue*.

I encourage you to:

✓ Rejuvenate your body
✓ Remember to be good to yourself

*IT'S ABOUT TIME* that you do!

*You deserve to relax and embrace your beauty.*

~~~~~~~~~~~~~

Now, earlier I talked about **brain fog** as one of the top menopause symptoms.

This mental spaciness can *seriously raise a woman's stress level*.

Jillian was stressed about brain fog, for example. So, in addition to having her take up yoga once or twice each week, I gave her some additional suggestions to reduce her brain fog, in order to combat stress.

Some of these, I've already mentioned in earlier parts of this book.

**But anything great is worth repeating!**

Everything that I coach is about *making diet and lifestyle changes*. So, if you want to **target brain fog** as a way to manage your menopause symptoms and lower your stress about them, **consider these ideas** as you develop an action plan.

### A. Decrease or Remove Wheat (Gluten)

**Eating the wrong food** is one of the biggest causes of long-term brain fog. It has been said that *no single food is worse* for causing and sustaining that fuzzy menopausal mind than <u>wheat gluten,</u> **and sensitivities**

to it. Gluten is a protein found in most grains, including wheat, rye and barley.

*What people eat does affect the brain*, particularly if they are allergic to gluten but do not realize it.

Food allergies can *disrupt the sensitive balance of hormones and chemicals* in the brain.

In Jillian's case, **avoiding gluten** directly improved her cognition, and lifted the brain fog so that she could think more clearly.

I've had other clients who found that getting off of gluten markedly stabilized their moods, increased their motor skills, and improved their concentration.

In his book Wheat Belly, Dr. William Davis writes about of how *wheat (gluten) can have a devastating impact on our cognitive faculties*, and how it *stimulates chronic brain fog.* He describes how weight loss, reduced fatigue, and superior mental clarity are the biggest benefits reported by patients who have stopped eating any wheat products, and have gone gluten-free.

### B. Stay Hydrated

When I first met with AnnaMaria about her mood swings and foggy moments, I encouraged her to **drink a lot more water** (preferably spring or distilled water). Water can **release the toxins** that accumulate in the intestinal tract. There are numerous studies that **link bowel toxicity directly to brain fog.** Water also helps to **flush the blood of metabolic waste products** that can travel to the brain and disrupt its functioning. When Suzanna began, every day, to drink half as many ounces of water as the amount of her body's weight (she weighs 128 pounds, so, 64 ounces), she felt that her mind clear right up.

### C. Socialize

**Staying social is crucial to brain health**. As you get older, you may be tempted to take the path that leads to the cushy sofa in front of the TV. Instead, put on your dancing shoes. **Get connected**. Start a book club, sign up for a class, volunteer, or throw a party!

### D. Feed Your Brain

When Lisa and Michelle changed their diet *to include more whole grains, fruits and vegetables, low-fat dairy, and lean protein,* a sharper mind was the wonderful side effect of such healthful eating. According to **The Menopause Book** by Pat Wingert and Barbara Kantrowitz, a healthy diet is also believed to *reduce your risk of dementia*.

~~~~~~~~

**Are you Still Wondering What to Eat for Superior Menopause Success?**

Let me tell you more about how I created the perfect menopause diet for Jillian, AnnaMaria, Michelle, and so many others, in the next chapter.

# -SIX-

# EATING PALEO for Menopause Health & Wellness

As I described in chapter 5, clients like Lizz began to build their perfect menopause diet by first **understanding how to manipulate their macronutrient breakdown**. Then, they **identified which phase they should adopt**. Finally, they **adjusted their diet plans to match their nutrition goals**.

When Jillian and Lizzette began to combat the menopausal changes in their metabolism and muscle mass by eating more cleanly and adding more activity, **they lost dozens of pounds**—but **never felt hungry**.

Yes, they discovered that you **can eat more and weigh less**.

PLUS, **the foods that I'm going to talk about in this chapter can actually taste delicious**.

But you have to know what you're doing.

After working with hundreds and hundreds of women, I have determined that ***the ideal diet solution for managing menopause includes adoption of the PALEO FRAMEWORK*** as your principle food plan of choice.

If you aren't yet familiar with the concept, the *Paleo Diet* consists of **foods that comprised the diet of early humans**. These "cave people" are known to have subsisted primarily on **wild plants and animal protein** that gave them great strength, plus immunity from various diseases that often challenge modern man.

I looked at the Paleo Diet from the perspective of menopause.

***How could it ameliorate or correlate to the symptoms that women describe most***:

- ▶ Night sweats
- ▶ Lost libido
- ▶ Poor sleep quality

- ▶ Weight gain
- ▶ Hot flashes
- ▶ Osteoporosis

I have discussed at length how *these symptoms are triggered by hormonal imbalance, especially the natural depletion of estrogen and progesterone*.

What the **Paleo Diet** offers to any woman who is in menopause is a **highly successful and proven way to** *prevent unwanted weight gain*, and to *facilitate healthy weight loss*, in conjunction with the exercise and stress-reduction components of the Menopause Success Triangle.

My very most current and groundbreaking success stories in menopause nutrition have shown me that the *Paleo Diet supplies your body with sufficient nutrients and energy to support a woman's daily activities, to prevent menopausal symptoms, to create stronger bones, to ward off infections, **and** to enhance a longer, healthier life*.

The key application of the Paleo Diet for Menopause is to **eliminate modern processed foods, sugar, dairy, and grains from your menu.**

Your diet should consist of:

▶ Meat (grass-fed only)
▶ Wild fish
▶ Eggs
▶ Vegetables (both leafy and tuberous)
▶ Oils
▶ Fruits
▶ Nuts

***These are the foods on which our original ancestors lived***.

What I have discovered is that the Paleo Diet has helped my clients to *regulate blood sugar*, which in turn has helped them to *regulate their hormones*. It has *increased the amount of magnesium* available to their body. It contains only *good, unrefined fats*. It is a simple, natural diet that effortlessly *rebalances the body's chemistry*. And it *really works to eliminate or ease many of the effects of menopause.*

The **natural weight loss** in my menopausal clients eating the Paleo Diet has given them a *new confidence, optimism,* and *feeling of wellbeing*. It's inspired them to **start new businesses, and take up new activities, even embark on risky and adventurous challenges**, like climbing Mt. Everest!

I highly recommend the <u>14-day Paleo Meal Plan</u> and <u>Paleo Diet Food List</u> at PaleoDietLifestyle.com, along with their cookbook—check it out on the banner below. It also has plenty of other helpful articles about diet tips and recipes.

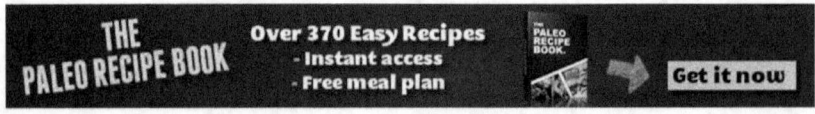

Dr. Loren Cordain is the founder of the Paleo Diet Movement. He's been seen on Dr. Oz, etc., and also has a highly resourceful <u>website about Paleo,</u> ThePaleoDiet.com. It covers the diet's **impact on various health and fitness conditions,** as well as **published research on the diet's success.**

Like I discussed in the nutrition section of chapter 5, *all successful menopause diets include plenty of:*

- *Fruits and vegetables*
- *Wholegrain carbs*
- *Healthy fats*
- *Lean protein*
- *CLEAN FOOD*

The successful menopause diet is organized around *eliminating processed foods and caffeine, limiting alcohol consumption, and sharply reducing the intake of processed sugar*.

Barbara had great success when she **broke up her daily meals into 5 smaller ones.** This was new for her: before the Menopause Success Triangle, she was used to eating one or two large meals each day.

Jillian's approach was to **get up from the table feeling not too full**—she was never too hungry, but she *avoided overeating* that way.

In working on an ideal menopause diet with Lizzette and Jillian, I showed them how their **liver and**

**gastrointestinal tracks** *were influencing their hormonal balance*, and how some of their symptoms seemed to tie to the fact that these important organs were falling out of whack.

Lizzette, for example, *loved her coffee in the morning*. And by itself, caffeine can be innocent enough. It even has some health-supporting properties!

BUT … when Lizzette and other peri-menopausal women drink it, they *trigger a hormonal imbalance in their intestines that also influences their liver*.

Lizzette also used to take **sugar and creamer** in her coffee, which further compounded the problem. The sugar *fed the development of yeast in her intestines*: yeast is **toxic when it becomes overabundant** and blocks the body from releasing used-up hormones, too.

Each part of this equation was *exacerbating Lizzette's cravings, mood swings, and fatigue*.

When she removed coffee from her diet, her hot flashes decreased, too, because caffeine triggers adrenaline, and adrenaline triggers a hot flash.

**Alcohol** is *processed in the liver* by the same *enzyme that processes estrogen*. So, when Jillian had her liver metabolize a glass of wine or a cocktail, it didn't have the capacity to process estrogen at the same time, the way she needed. She *noticed this dip in her estrogen processing every time that she had a drink:* it **triggered her night sweats**, and sometimes **hot flashes**, too.

AnnaMaria and Michelle used to *crave the same types of processed foods* that they gobbled up when they were PMS-ing: **potato chips, doughnuts, sugary breakfast cereals, soda, and juices** laden with sugar.

*Each one of these treats **has to *FALL OFF THE LIST*** of things to feed your body during menopause.*

In their place, I had these women begin to eat more items *from a different list*. The "My Body is Begging for These" List!

> ▶ *Almonds*
> ▶ *Soy beans*
> ▶ *Legumes*
> ▶ *Carrots*
> ▶ *Broccoli*
> ▶ *Melons*
> ▶ *Cantaloupes*
> ▶ *Grapes*

I convinced AnnaMaria that she *couldn't have enough fresh fruit in her diet, <u>ever</u>!*

Michelle thought that she just **didn't have time to eat all of the veggies** she needed. So, she takes a vegetable juice with her when she is on the move.

Just by eating more vegetables and fruits over seven days, the *two of them noticed a marked difference* in the way they felt!

When I talked to Jillian about her diet, it was clear that she also **needed more** *fiber* **in her diet**. She replaced sugary breakfast cereal with oatmeal or fiber cereal on most mornings, and since she loves bread, she still has a little toast, but tries to make it **wheat or bran** rather than a processed, white refined-flour product.

Barbara and I came up with a list of **alternatives for the fried and processed foods** that had been in her diet during her weight gain. For instance, she *replaced white pasta with wheat pasta,* and *white potatoes with sweet potatoes*. Then, she started to *eat numerous little meals* throughout her day, and everything in moderation.

These little tweaks made a huge difference, and helped her to **lose 22 pounds in 14 weeks**.

AnnaMaria was open to starting her menopause diet reset with a cleanse. I'm **not a fan of cleanses in the traditional sense**—the typical "pop-a-pill" and spend all day on the toilet-type. Those cleanses **focus on the WRONG thing**.

They want you to believe that, by buying bottles of their herbal concoctions and supplements, or by drinking gallons of "spicy lemonade," you'll be able to lose weight and feel more alive than ever. Although these products may show quick results, they *rarely lead to lasting change*. What good is it to lose 20 pounds in two weeks, only to pack it right back on again after your detox is complete, when you revert to your old ways of eating?

**I want quick AND lasting change for you.**

I want you to *enjoy incredible vitality, and a body that you can feel proud* of, not just for a few days but FOREVER.

So, here are **3 healthy cleansing strategies** that AnnaMaria and others of my clients adopted, based on their making small adjustments to the most important thing that you do each day.

## #1 - Get Your AM Drink On

Yes, that's right ... I had AnnaMaria **_drink, first thing in the morning._** But it was **WATER.** And lots of it. I had her start each day with **ONE LITER** of water before ingesting anything else.

**_Why?_**

Two reasons...

First, she and everyone else **_lose a lot of water during sleep through their breathing._** Therefore, <u>rehydrating</u> is an important thing to do, when you wake up.

Second, since a person is immobile during sleep, **_toxins, produced by the body which need to be excreted_**, **_build up_** in the liver. Drinking water in the morning can help you to <u>move those toxins</u> out of your system swiftly, into your urine and stool.

<u>Bonus tip:</u> *Add a squeeze of lemon* to your morning water. Lemon stimulates gall bladder contractions, which facilitate the removal of those

stored toxins. Lemon also awakens the rest of your digestive tract so that you'll find yourself hopping on the toilet quicker than by drinking a morning coffee, and it also balances your alkaline pH, so that antibiotics and food don't stain your teeth.

## #2 - Go Green and Enjoy a Liquid Lunch

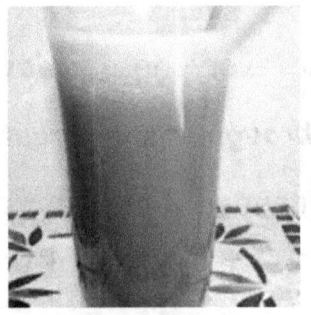

If I were to give you ONE strategy that could improve your body and health dramatically, it would be to **add more greens into your diet**. As I convinced Michelle, the easiest way to do that is by liquefying them.

Because, let's be honest ... Unless you're a cow grazing the pasture, you're *most likely not going to eat grasses and leafy greens all day long*. But you can certainly throw greens like kale, parsley, Swiss chard, lettuce, and green powder into a blender, right?

The ***power of green vegetables lies in their incredibly*** *high levels of vitamins, minerals, and disease-fighting phytonutrients.*

Greens are also the major source of alkalinity within our food supply. Without getting too technical here, just realize that, when your body is too acidic (from eating grains, sugar, salt, and animal products), it becomes prone to sickness, disease, and lethargy.

By eating more vegetables, especially greens, you can **restore the natural alkaline pH that your blood requires** for optimal health.

Here's my go-to lunchtime smoothie that I know you'll enjoy, too:

1 head of kale, Swiss chard, or dark green lettuce

½ handful of cilantro

1 apple

1 pear

1 banana

Juice of ½ lime

500 ml of water

Throw everything into a blender, and you'll get about 1 liter of cleansing power that tastes amazing!

### #3 - Remove Common Congesting and Allergenic Foods (at least temporarily)

As I discussed with Jillian, Lizzette, and AnnaMaria, *foods like sugar, caffeine, and alcohol are the obvious ones to scratch* off the list when you cleanse.

But not many people realize that *foods like corn, soy, grains, and most animal products (especially dairy) are very congesting*, and they tax your digestive and immune systems, as well.

My client Deborah found that, when she ate these "allergenic" foods on a regular basis, her immune system *identified their proteins as foreign invaders*, which **stimulated inflammation** throughout her body.

She suffered from **excess mucus and congestion**, in addition to major **dips in her daily energy**.

So I had her try this technique.

I really recommend that you experiment with it, too.

She *removed all of those foods* from her diet for a few days. Then, once she noticed that she had more energy, less congestion, and better bowel movements, plus had already begun to shed needless fat, she began to *add them back into her diet one at a time*, and kept a journal about their effects on her body.

She was shocked! She is OK with lean meat and low-fat yogurt, but had to find great alternatives to corn, sugar, and soy. *Now, she feels great with whatever she eats.*

## Where Can I Start with This type of Cleanse?

Here is the simple one-day meal plan that I gave to AnnaMaria. She discovered right away *how delicious a*

***proper "food-based" cleanse can be*** … And adapted it to carry her through an entire week!

## Breakfast: Coconut Blue-Cranberry Smoothie

    1 cup fresh or frozen blueberries
    1/4 cup fresh or frozen whole cranberries
    250ml coconut milk
    250ml water

## Lunch: Leek and Onion Soup

    3 leek stalks
    1 large onion
    5 garlic cloves, minced
    5 stalks celery, juiced
    1 carrot, juiced
    2 Tbsp Braggs Liquid Aminos to taste
    1 Tbsp fresh rosemary, chopped
    2 Tbsp olive oil (optional)
    4 cups water
    Fresh ground black pepper to taste

<u>Dinner</u>: Roasted Veggie and Quinoa Perfection

> 1 cup quinoa
>
> 2 cups water
>
> 2 small zucchinis, chopped
>
> 1 medium carrot, chopped
>
> 1 small red onion, chopped
>
> 2 Tbsp coconut oil
>
> 1 sweet potato, peeled and chopped
>
> 1 yellow squash, peeled and chopped
>
> Juice of one fresh lemon
>
> Sea salt to taste

1. Roast chopped vegetables in the oven at 300°F until tender.

2. Bring the quinoa and water to a boil in a medium pot, then reduce the heat to a simmer and let cook for 10-12 minutes, or until water is absorbed and quinoa is fluffy.

3. Place bed of quinoa on plate and surround or top with roasted vegetables, a splash of fresh lemon juice, and sea salt to taste.

~~~~~~~~

I hope that these ideas ***get your taste buds sizzling***!

Cleansing is **absolutely critical** to your health (since we're all way too toxic). But it *doesn't have to revolve around crazy herbal supplements*.

Instead, it can <u>and should</u> be based on **eating clean whole foods.** That's the only way you can achieve quick and long-lasting results.

After all, y*ou're improving your dietary habits one day at a time*—and improving your daily habits is what counts in the long run.

## How about the RAW FOOD Idea?

Eating **raw foods** is *not a menopause diet that works for everyone*, but I have seen plenty of research on its merits. Plus, I had personal success with Susanne and Kasi, who adopted a *raw food diet in order to balance out the side effects of their hormonal imbalances* that were caused by menopause.

Raw vegetables are rich in enzymes and phyto-estrogens, which can restore your hormonal system to a necessary and healthy balance.

Susanne didn't go totally raw

Kasi, on the other hand, gave it a try and really enjoyed it.

Both of them *began by eating more nicely cleaned, fresh vegetables with every meal*.

They also **stayed away from processed foods**, and **minimized the amounts of cooked food** in their daily diet, along with food that had been **over-heated**. They found **loads of raw food salad recipes** to choose from on the internet

I really like Yuri's Elkaim's Eating For Energy Program. Check it out!

∼∼∼∼∼∼∼∼

OKAY, How about SOY?...

Before we end this chapter on **Eating Paleo for Menopause Health and Wellness,** I'd like to bring up the *subject of SOY*.

My clients Lisa and Lizz were looking for *a natural approach to their menopausal symptoms—hot flashes, night sweats, and the heat rage*. They wanted to try **using soy products as a nutritional fire extinguisher,**

I shared with them *both sides of the debate* around this strategy.

The **soy bean** is *one of the most potent sources of phytoestrogens* that has been found in the "natural world." Many food stores now carry a wide array of soy products, from milk and cheese, to soy chorizo and chocolate pudding. Vegetarians use it as an alternative to meat. Tofu, a common ingredient in Asian cuisine, is a curd made from soy milk.

**Soy beans are potent isoflavones**, like other beans (navy, pinto or kidney beans, chick peas or garbanzo beans, lentils and peanuts). **Soy derivatives** like soy milk, whole soybeans (edamame), miso, and soy yogurt are also **isoflavones**.

In Asian countries, soy is a dietary staple, and has helped women there to have fewer hot flashes than women in the U.S.

But, when **studies have looked closely at soy's effects on menopausal symptoms,** the results have been mixed.

In Europe, particularly in Italy, soy was connected with a **45% reduction in the hot flashes** of women who consumed soy protein, compared to a 30% improvement in the placebo group.

But … for every positive study, **there has been another one that shows little or no benefits** that correlate to the consumption of soy.

In March 2002, *The Journal of Obstetrics & Gynecology* published research on menopausal women who took a daily dose of 100 mg of **soy isoflavones** (an estrogen-like constituent of soy that appears to be the key ingredient for easing hot flashes). These women experienced a **significant** *decline in their menopausal symptoms, including hot flashes, mood swings, and sleep difficulties.*

But in another study in 2002 at Tufts University, researchers found that, after three months of soy supplementation, **women had no more relief from hot flashes than another group taking a placebo** (dummy) pill!

Some physicians such as Machelle Seibel, MD and Mary Hardy, MD have **found positive connections**. They believe that good data now indicates that **soy can reduce both the frequency and intensity of hot flashes during menopause**. Others have found that reducing hot flashes with soy to 50% isn't enough. They strive to eliminate this particular symptom completely.

Lisa and Lizz were **thrilled to reduce their hot flashes by some percentage** through adding more soy and other isoflavones to their diets.

Lisa definitely slept better than before, and felt more able to cope.

Both she and Lizz added soy to their diets in combination with a healthier, more Paleo-oriented overall diet, natural supplements, and exercise, however.

Together*, these lifestyle changes had a huge impact on reducing their symptoms of hot flashes and night sweats*.

Incorporating soy into the diet **has not worked for everyone** whom I coach. So I always recommend that you **weigh the pros and cons of soy**, the same as you would HRT.

Discover **what really works for you**.

Don't try any of these strategies as a "quick fix": it is really important to be patient, and give all new diets and exercise plans a fair chance to work for you.

And while soy may not have a complete effect on your menopausal symptoms like hot flashes, that is not the most important reason to take soy. **The heart-and bone-strengthening benefits are also important!** For example, there is such strong evidence now that **soy can reduce blood cholesterol levels** that the FDA permits this claim on food labels.

If you want to give soy a try, most experts recommend **consuming one to two servings per day,** which translates to taking *about 25 to 50 mg* of isoflavones. If you don't experience any benefit from two servings of soy, then **try adding a third**, or the equivalent as a supplement.

If you aren't a fan of naturally-based soy foods, then *soy supplements—most of which contain 25 mg of isoflavones per pill—are available at health-food stores*.

# -SEVEN-

## To Supplement or NOT To Supplement: THAT IS THE QUESTION

I think that *food should be thy medicine.*

However ... **SUPPLEMENTATION** can *help women fill in some missing pieces in their daily diet*.

There is a **lively debate about the viability of natural and medicinal approaches to various menopause symptoms.**

**HRT (hormone therapy)** involves supplementing a woman's key reproductive hormones with *medicines that include estrogen and progestin (artificial progesterone)*. A great deal of research now <u>**recommends against HRT**</u> because of its association with increased risk for uterine and breast cancer.

So, *natural therapies have become more popular.*

Many of the women that I coach have seen improvements in body and mind after adding **natural therapies and supplements** to their lives.

Some of my clients have incorporated **new vitamins, minerals, herbs, and other supplements** into their nutrition plan. They use them to *address select symptoms*, *support their weight loss efforts*, and/or *enhance their overall health*.

Here are ***some of their success stories,*** but, as you consider them, also please ***REMEMBER***—one woman may ***need vitamin E*** to minimize her hot flashes. Another may want to ***try gingko to enhance her mental clarity,*** etc.

**First and foremost: supplementation is very personal**.

There is some great research and information available on natural remedies at the moment. Personally, I've found that supplementation contributes best to the Menopause Success Triangle after an initial ***analysis of a woman's blood chemistry***, and then through the ***addition of and experimentation with select products and various doses***.

## PRODUCTS

Susanne, Barbara, and Nadi each tried ***adding to their diets the six vitamins and minerals*** that I call the "Magic Six."

They wanted to feel better and lose weight. I've concluded that ***every woman should take these six vitamins and minerals***, at minimum, as soon as they begin peri-menopause.

*A. Vitamin C:* Nadi was already taking vitamin C during the winter time in order to ***boost her immune system and fight off colds***. When she started to work out for the first time at 44, however, she decided to **increase her dose to 3,000 mg** daily, because I showed her how Vitamin C ***helps to rebuild tired muscles and repair wounds***. She did this through combining a supplement with an increase in her diet of foods like citrus fruits, kale, broccoli, and Brussels sprouts.

B. *Vitamin D* helps the body to **absorb calcium**, a crucial mineral that a woman's body loses as she gets older. Barbara's mother had osteoporosis, so when she learned that Vitamin D is also good for the bones, she increased her intake of **salmon and tuna, eggs and soy milk**. She also allowed her skin to **absorb twenty minutes of sunshine** every day that she could get outside, and she added 2,500 IUs daily in supplement form.

C. *Fish Oils:* Susanne, like many women going through menopause, was *at risk for heart disease*. Fish oil is an Omega-3 fatty acid, the sort best known to ***lower the incidence of heart disease.*** In the sources section that comes later in this chapter, I recommend a high-density Omega-3 product that comes from **krill**; you may want to consider taking it, too. *If you currently take any sort of blood thinners, however, you* *should consult your doctor first before taking fish oil* supplements or increasing your intake of seafood fats.

*D. Flax Seeds:* these little golden seeds are **packed with antioxidants and omega-3s, plus lignans** (a source of plant estrogen) and **fiber.** They are a good alternative to eating fish or taking fish oil supplements, and while they are healthy for you to eat at any time, they seem ***better at minimizing peri-menopausal symptoms*** rather than post-menopausal hot flashes. Be very careful that the seeds, oil, or ground powder of flax are **kept refrigerated and used quickly**: flaxseeds spoil rapidly, and rancid ones bring on a toxicity that can make you feel horrible.

*E. Calcium:* Barbara also took supplemental calcium in order to *counter the bone loss* ***that often accompanies a decrease in estrogen.*** She also took vitamin D and magnesium to **ensure that her calcium was absorbed well**, and she also **rotated the sources** of her calcium supplements every few months to prevent the development of any intolerance or lowered sensitivity. (Magnesium is also known as "nature's tranquilizer," so Barbara found that it helped her with her irritability and other mood changes, as well.)

*F. Black Cohosh & St. John's Wort:* **Black Cohosh** is one of nature's secret weapons against symptoms of menopause. Nadi and AnnaMaria all found that it had a strong impact on reducing their hot flashes and depression. Denise and Lisa combined it with the herb **St. John's Wort** in a tincture that had a marked effect on their mood swings, and greatly lessened their irritability.

For clients like Lizzette and Lizz who were struggling with hot flashes and night sweats, I recommended that they try, in addition to black cohosh, these three supplements:

*G. Bioflavonoids:* these are low-toxicity plant compounds with ***high anti-oxidant properties*** that help you not just with your hot flashes and hormone regulation, but they ward off cancer tumors, as well. **Citrus fruits and berries, onions**, and **green or white tea** are popular sources of bioflavonoids. So is **dark chocolate**, which my clients have decided is *well worth a try* as a tasty, healthy addition to their diet. (In moderation, and with low sugar, though!)

*H. Vitamin E:* this supplement, which comes in oil form, is a *unique antioxidant* that really helps to maintain a woman's skin and hair while also protecting her heart from arteriosclerosis. Denise took Vitamin E when she discovered that *vaginal dryness* was affecting her healthy sexuality. She both ate more **wheat germ, sunflower seeds**, and **almonds**, in order to be sure she took **400 IUs** each day of vitamin E, **AND** she used the E oil *topically on her skin and vagina.*

*I. Soy isoflavones:* as I mentioned in chapter 6, Lizz found relief from her hot flashes by *adding soy to her diet* on a regular basis. Isoflavones are a component of soy and other plants that have phytoestrogenic properties, so their naturally-occurring hormones protect a woman's body from the nefarious effects of estrogen while they balance your internal hormonal levels. In addition to **soy** and **flaxseed**s, other isoflavones **include hops, dandelion, red clover, sage,** and **alfalfa.**

Kasi decided to ***add some bio-identical estrogen*****, oestradiol cream**, to her health profile, so, in order to protect herself from adverse effects of estrogen, she also takes the **powerful isoflavone diindolylmethane (DIM)**. *DIM* is ***found in cruciferous vegetables*** including broccoli, cauliflower, cabbage, and Brussels sprouts, and is readily available in supplement form. AnnaMaria had success balancing her own glandular system and increasing her stamina by taking *Mexican wild yam* (Dioscorea villosa). It isn't a phytoestrogen but ***contains a phytonutrient that is a precursor for*** *progesterone.* She found that using the yam cream also *decreased the severity of her hot flashes.*

Clients like Deborah and Susanne also had success with lowering their stress and increasing their relaxation by supplementing their healthy diet, exercise, and meditation with a few natural vitamins and herbs.

*J. B Vitamins:* these are called **the "stress" vitamins**, because they **help so much when you feel anxious, tense, and irritable**. Suzanna increased her dosage of B's in supplement form, and found that she had more patience and concentration. I recommended to Lisa that she, too, take a good B-complex supplement in order to give her adrenal glands a rest; she found that the vitamins helped to increase her energy levels, too.

*K. Chamomile, valerian & kava root:* Deborah added a supplement to her bedtime routine that included **kava kava, valerian root**, and **passiflora**. She found that it helped to calm her mind tremendously. Valerian also helped to minimize Kasi's occasional feelings of anxiety—but she was careful *not to combine it with alcohol*. Susanne has been **drinking chamomile tea** in the evenings, which has lowered her stress levels, as well.

*L. Lavender oil:* this lovely-smelling plant extract has been *used as a relaxant for centuries*. AnnaMaria puts a **few drops in a warm bath** after a stressful day, while Michelle **freshens her pillow** with a little oil whenever she feels anxious, or wants to ensure more restful sleep. You can even put a **dab on your chest** and on each wrist, if you need to de-stress in the middle of a busy day.

~~~~~~~~~

In the next section I recommend some powerful products that have provided myriad benefits for clients that I coach. Many of the menopausal women in my practice come to me with concerns about weight loss and belly fat, so these last two stand-alone supplements are natural products that helped Lizzette, Barbara and Jillian *amp up their fat-burning metabolism and shed pounds fast.*

*M. Raspberry Ketones:* the compound that gives raspberries that delicious smell has also been called *a "fat burner in a bottle."* It regulates *adiponectin*, which is a protein that the body uses to *regulate metabolism*. So raspberry ketone causes the fat in your cells to break down more effectively, and helps the body burn fat faster. Lizzette found that taking this supplement in conjunction with exercise and a whole-food diet also gave her extra energy.

*N. Brown seaweed fucoxanthin:* Fucoxanthin is a *carotenoid found in edible brown seaweed*, and extracts have been linked in some studies with *weight loss, particularly for abdominal fat.* Some research has shown that it helps "bad" white adipose fat mimic "good" brown fat, which burns energy rather than stores it. It is also a powerful anti-oxidant that fights inflammation.

*O. Caffeine, Green Tea, Cinnamon, and Other Metabolism Boosters:* Caffeine is a stimulant. Studies show that it can boost your metabolism a bit, but also please remember its **correlation to sleep issues and stress.** Some women become more sensitive to the insomniac effects of caffeine in menopause, while others who could never take a sip of coffee during their reproductive years come to find that they can enjoy coffee or espresso, as they age.

There is an ***antioxidant in green tea and green coffee*** called ***EGCG*** that has **also been linked to speeding metabolism.** Another natural metabolism booster is **cinnamon**, which I ***think is great.*** Recent health advocates also support **calcium** and a group of fatty acids known as **CLA (conjugated linoleic acid)** for their ability to boost metabolism.

## SUPPLEMENT RESOURCES & VENDORS

When I meet with clients and analyze the relationship between their nutrition plans and the symptoms that they are experiencing, I ***always recommend a combination of the minerals and herbs*** mentioned above.

The following are my **top six** supplement recommendations, along with explanations for how they work. I also ***embed web links*** to where you can find, read more about, and buy them.

(The products at Pro-grade can be ordered through the product listing on the left-hand side of the landing page. You can find even more extensive explanations on each product there, too, along with some benefit videos, as well.)

1. <u>Prograde ® EFA Icon Krill Oil</u>: (found at <u>www.metaburnnutrition.com</u>) this is a top-grade omega-3 supplement that can offer you ***a revolutionary and quantum improvement for your***

*health*. **Krill oil** is very different than regular fish oil, and very hard to get because krill are small crustaceans found only in the Southern Ocean and Antarctic Ocean.

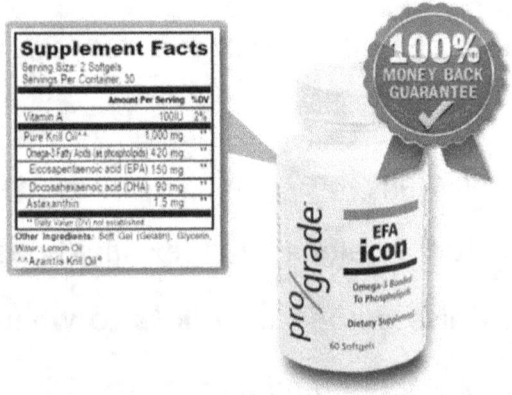

The reason that I like this product is because its ***antioxidant power is 297 times greater than vitamin A or E,*** and **47 times greater than regular fish oil**! It also includes ***astaxanthin,*** which readily crosses the blood-brain barrier, so that your **brain is protected and stimulated** during menopause. My clients who take EFA Icon have found that it helps them to have a better mood, better memory and clearer thinking. This krill oil product also includes ***phospholipids*** that filter toxins, and has ***no fishy after-taste or acid reflux*** that often bothers women who take regular fish oil supplements.

2.    Longevity    Anti-Aging    Formula:    (at metaburnnutrition.com)

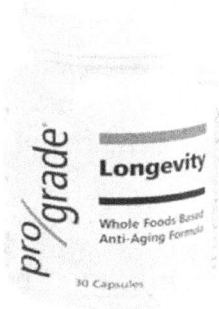

As we age, our healthy cells are constantly vulnerable to free radicals that try to damage them and bring on disease. ***Free radicals are fed by stress, processed foods, air pollutants, and the aging process***, even when we follow a healthy diet and exercise program. The **only thing that combats free radicals is anti-oxidants**. I find that this Prograde® LONGEVITY formula pours the most effective anti-aging, health-improving nutrients into one tiny

**capsule**. Clinical studies have shown that it can help to lower blood pressure, strengthen your nervous system, improve your retinas, detoxify the body, reduce pain, strengthen the heart, **and** prevent strokes. Most important, these nutrients can slow the aging process in both body and brain.

LONGEVITY includes the *same antioxidants as 459 fresh blueberries, plus açaí berry, more anthocyanins than red wine, green tea extract, polyphenols, pomegranate and wolfberry extract, and a new nutrient called CoffeeBerry®* that has also been shown in recent studies to help ease joint pain, lower cholesterol, reduce tooth decay and gum disease, fight allergies by blocking histamine and IgE (immunoglobulin E), fend off infection, prevent wrinkles that come from cell oxidation, and improve memory. I really think that your results from this product are guaranteed to be terrific!

### 3. Pro-X10™ Advanced Probiotic and GI Health

<u>Formula:</u> (found at menopause.biotrust.com)

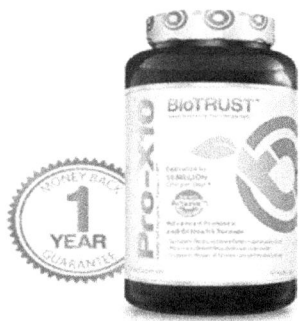

I think that you can ***accelerate fat loss and drastically improve your health by eating "friendly" bacteria***. Our gastrointestinal track does so much more than just digest food. It is also a "**second brain,**" and **home to 80% of your immune system** through 100 trillion living bacteria.

**Supporting the ratio of good to bad bacteria is finally being recognized as a key to our health *and* to our fat-loss efforts.**

When a woman's intestinal bacteria is out of balance, she experiences gas and bloating; constipation and/or diarrhea; fatigue; headaches; and sugar cravings, especially for heavily refined carbs—the very same symptoms that have plagued so many women during menopause!

The ideal healthy ratio of "good" to "bad" bacteria is 85% to 15%, or 9 to 1. Unfortunately, due to lifestyle and environmental factors, the **vast majority of the population is severely lacking when it comes to good probiotic bacteria**, which throws their gut flora ratio completely out of whack. So, unless you maintain a 100% organic diet, completely avoid all sugar, and lock yourself in the house with only the purest of air for 24 hours a day, 7 days a week, it is **almost certain that your gut flora balance is suffering,** and will continue to do so unless you are proactive about correcting it.

I recommend a carefully researched product like Pro-X10™, because it **ensures live probiotics that stay active all the way to your intestine**. Pro-X10 uses a cutting-edge, patented microencapsulation technology to deliver a potent supplement to support your gut health, and more. Check it out at the website menopause.biotrust.com!

4. **Pro/Grade Protein Powder:** (find at MetaburnNutrition.com)

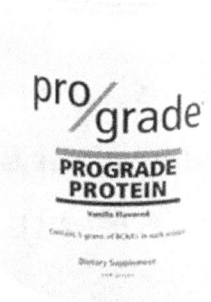

Sometimes you may want to **supplement your meal or snack with a high-quality protein shake**. For two reasons, I recommend Pro-Grade's cutting-edge protein powder to clients that are working on weight loss:

▶ Each serving has 24 grams of proteins that boost your metabolism
▶ The Pro-Grade formulation signals the brain, so that you feel full longer.

Studies have shown that proteins like Pro-Grade's, which are **rich in** leucine, **promote fat loss while preserving your lean muscle tissue**. They help to stabilize your blood glucose levels by slowing down glucose absorption; when insulin levels are lower, it is easier for your body to burn fat. And their whey protein stimulates the **release of two hormones that suppress the appetite:** cholecystokinin **(CCK) and glucagon-like** peptide-**1** **(GLP-1).** The whey protein also helps you to feel fuller than casein (the other protein in milk), so this product makes for great mid-day snack.

5. **VG-25+ Multivitamin**: (available at MetaburnNutrition.com)

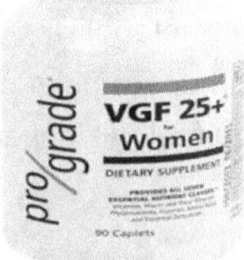

I am a huge proponent of a healthy diet full of fresh fruits and vegetables for many reasons. But I have had clients express *how hard it can be to get all of the nutrients and vitamins that they need every day*.

I researched multi-vitamin/multi-mineral products, and really love Pro-Grade's V-25+ because it is **specifically formulated for women, to support their hormone balance**. This product includes the concentrates of 25 whole vegetables, greens and fruits, so, it promotes fat burning, helps to boost energy levels and moods, improves my clients' sleep quality, and has reduced their stress levels. I have also seen women who take this supplement grow stronger nails and shinier hair. And none of my clients have complained that this product upsets their stomach, like some multi-vitamins do. VGF 25+ for Women provides *whole food-based nutrition that keeps your body's system running like a well-oiled machine*!

6. <u>Green Mix – Genesis</u>: **(available at MetaburnNutrition.com)**

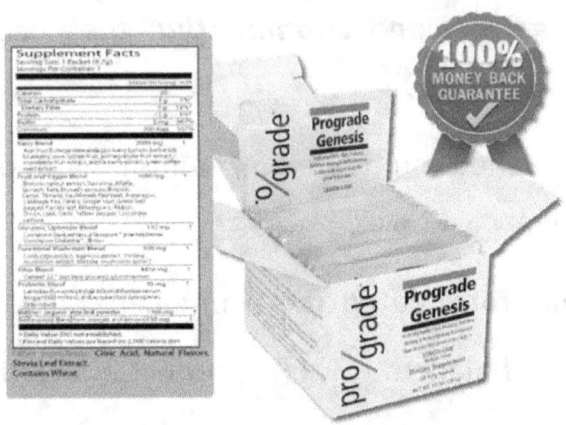

I love this greens superfood supplement, and think that it is ***one of the best detoxing formulas on the market***. It's called GENESIS, and helps to ***ensure that you have the support that you need to stay well, look good, lower inflammation, and even lose a few pounds in the process***! I have my clients start their day with GENESIS because it helps their bodies to ***maximize the nutritional benefits of the foods*** that they eat throughout the day.

GENESIS **tackles free-radicals**, those unstable molecules that are missing an electron. It supports your body's free-radical defense system to fight off sickness and disease, and it dampens the flames of inflammation that irritate joints and provoke discomfort.

~~~~~~~~

Supplementation is a great resource. Fortunately, it is at your disposal as you develop your personal menopause success program.

You can dive in to these tips, discuss them with your doctor or coach, and evaluate how each vitamin or supplement can support your great health and well-being.

***Don't be overwhelmed*** by the possibilities and prescriptions. These are **just great tools,** readily available, to **help you feel, look, and perform better** as you age, and as you continue to define your own menopausal self!

# -EIGHT-

# 21 TIPS FOR SUCCESS

I agree with so many experts on this fact: *a positive new direction can be established, or a bad habit can be broken, in JUST 21 DAYS.*

That is, provided that you **focus** on that change with your **full intention.**

I love to give my clients **concrete steps** that they can take in order to make a difference in their lives. I want to help each one of them—and you, too—achieve *all of your goals for wellbeing, happiness, and fulfillment*.

As you work through a new diet and exercise plan like Lizz and Barbara did, and as you add yoga and meditation to your day in order to lower stress like Jillian and Michelle did, I want to offer you **21 more tips** that support a positive change in your menopause lifestyle.

*Try one each week*.

Some of them complement and *enhance your new nutrition plan*. Some will maximize your *success at new exercise and activities.* Others are great for *countering the stressors of brain fog* and other mindsets that challenge your motivation and energy.

1. Don't skip meals & Eat on a schedule. This is especially important when it comes to breakfast. WHY? Because breakfast will **boost your metabolism for the rest of the day.** Eat a **good, healthy breakfast**. When you skip a meal, your metabolism slows down, and your body's natural defenses take over. It's that "famine effect," albeit on a micro-level. But *a hungry body without breakfast really does start to store fat and save it for fuel* when needed. So, think of breakfast as one of your metabolism boosters, and eat. Remember, **fat loss** is what you're

aiming for. You will always **burn more fat when your metabolism is working** at its best.

Now, breakfast **does not have to be a huge meal.** You could eat just a **quick bowl of cereal** or a **yogurt**. Beat an **egg** with salt and pepper and pop it into the microwave for a minute and a half, even top it with a little **grated cheese**. Whatever you do, start your day right with a healthy diet, and eat breakfast.

Then, *eat smaller amounts at each of your 5-6 meals* every day. I've found that to be <u>an excellent strategy for any menopausal nutrition plan</u>.

*REPLACE The Idea of Eating *Only Breakfast, Lunch and Dinner.**

With a meal plan, the process becomes easier. Map out your breakfast, snack, lunch, afternoon snack, dinner, and after-dinner snack—even include in the plan where you want to drink your 64 ounces of water daily.

Think about it as **six small meals every three hours or so, <u>starting with breakfast!</u>**

2. Avoid processed foods, which often contain high levels of fat and sugar. **Fresh fruit and vegetables**, and **whole grains**, along with **healthy fats** and **protein** at each meal, are the best things to eat for people who are trying to lose weight, and to build lean muscle as a metabolism-booster. Investigate some amazing alternatives at the <u>Paleo Lifestyle and Recipe Book site.</u>

3. Make sure that you get enough sleep. Many adults manage on six hours of sleep every night, but this leads to a reduced metabolism and weight gain, over time. The Royal College of Psychiatrists' advice on getting a good night's sleep is to *go to bed and get up in the morning at the same time every day; avoid naps* during

the day; and *have a hot bath before bed* (as hot as you can bear without scalding yourself) for at least 20 minutes.

4. **Instead of using butter in your cooking, use coconut or olive oil,** which are both much healthier types of fat.

5. **Don't eat within three hours** of going to bed. Consider that, when you lay out your plan.

This doesn't mean that you can't enjoy going out to restaurants!

But *think about eating* two-course meals. Even if you have a sweet tooth, **skip dessert** as often as you can. Your post-menopausal body cannot handle the excess sugar, and converts it into fat for later use. Sugar-rich food is the primary reason for weight gain in women.

A **dessert once a week**, or indulging yourself **only** when you are out at **a social event,** is ideal.

Every time that you feel the urge for dessert, try *scooping spoonsful of cold yogurt*. It feels like a dessert, and causes no harm to your body. And here's an additional tip: **when you eat out**, *take half of the serving home for a snack the next day.*

6. Clear out the bad stuff. Replace it with the good stuff. Are there things in your pantry that you need to donate to a relative or a food bank?

Call a couple of your close friends, and enlist them to *clean out your kitchen of all unhealthy food items*. These include all of those **cans of sugar-rich sodas, fried chips,** and any other processed or packaged food like **cookies, cakes, candy**, and **potato chips**. Unless and until you have checked the calorie content and ingredients in a particular food item, *Discard It.* **ANYTHING WHITE MUST GO!** (That means white pasta, sugar, potatoes, and flour.) Try to do this on a full stomach, so you're not tempted to eat those potato chips, instead of toss them!

*THEN* ... **get addicted to fruits**—they are so good for your body. Every time that you have hunger pangs between meals, ***grab an apple or a banana*** to satisfy your need, or scoop out the tender flesh of a kiwi.

***Stock your refrigerator with fruits, and fill your pantry with nuts and dried fruit.*** Keep a bowl of almonds or dried apricots on your work desk or dining table. They are rich sources of the nutrients and enzymes that are most essential for your body.

7. **Make a food list:** This should be easy to do when you begin to replace any white foods in your life with brown and colorful, non-processed goodies.

   Start your list with **whole-wheat pasta and flour, brown rice, grapes, banana, strawberries, melons,** (any fruit that is in season and that you love), and **vegetables** that you can eat within a few days. Include **flaxseeds** or flaxseed oil on the list, too, so that you can include 2 tablespoons in your smoothie or salad dressing every day to boost your metabolism. When it comes to fruits and vegetables, *there are no limits* on your list.

8. **Protein with Every Meal:** Another great metabolism-boosting trick is to eat **lots of protein**. By adding protein to every meal, you will *improve your lean muscle mass*. The more lean muscle that you have in your body, the higher your **BMR** will be. Because of the thermic effect of food, and how quickly insulin is released into the body after you consume it, you need to *have a good, solid, clean protein with every meal*—a **piece of chicken or fish, an egg or some nuts**—in order to **slow down the thermal process** when you eat.

Don't worry! I'm not saying that you have to bulk up and become a body builder. Just **focus on eating the right foods**. By adding protein to every meal, you will help to fuel your body with muscle. Protein can be found in a variety of foods from many different food groups. **Red meat**, of course, is the first thing that comes to mind. But foods like **turkey or chicken, cottage cheese, fish** and **egg whites** are other **great sources of protein**.

~~~~~~~~~

As you increase your daily and weekly activity for a more vibrant menopause lifestyle, and as you develop a personal exercise plan that challenges and inspires you, consider these tips:

9. **Choose an exercise program and activities that you enjoy**, so that you will stick to them. And **change it up.** If you are following my 21-day Menopause Success Triangle Workout Plan,

*shuffle the order* when you start it a second or third time. Also, try *different types of aerobic activities* like jazz or hip-hop dance, maybe biking or cross-country skiing. And think about gardening as one of your strength-building activities.

10. **Find an accountability partner**, someone who will exercise with you so that you stay motivated. Sometimes you may feel too tired to squeeze in your workout, but *your partner can remind* you that regular exercise makes you feel less tired in the long run, and increases your energy and metabolism, all of which work together to help keep your weight down.

A single 15-minute walk can *give you an energy boost.* Morning exercise is the best. Start with a small amount of exercise together, and then build up your physical activity gradually over weeks and months until you reach the recommended goal of 30 minutes to an hour each day of moderate-intensity aerobic exercise like cycling or fast walking, combined with strength-training exercises that help to maintain muscle mass.

11. **Wear comfortable clothing so that you don't get overheated**. Sweat, but don't swelter! Check out our Resource List, Chapter 10, for ***great, wicking workout clothes that keep you cool***. And include on that list a ***terrific, supportive pair of sneakers***. Nike and others have cross-trainers that are very light and flexible, and also good for walking/running as though you're barefoot. Other brands have lots of ankle support, if you're concerned about tweaking your tendons. Try the various shoes on and jump around the store a little; and also, ***replace them every few hundred miles***!

12. **Pick a start date.** I love this affirmation by Tony Robbins: ***"A real decision is measured by the fact that you've taken a new action. If there's no action, you haven't truly decided."***

    Or, as Benjamin Franklin said, *"If you fail to plan, you plan to fail."*

13. **Always talk to your doctor** about a new exercise program before beginning. And **keep a journal** of what you do, what you eat, along any questions or pains that arise, so that you can check in on them, plus discuss them with your trainer or coach. We *want* to remember, but ***writing it down makes it so much easier!*** And writing is a powerful tool that can help you to express how you are feeling throughout your menopause-lifestyle reset journey.

14. **Drink more water:** I like to repeat this tip because it affects so many things. And it ***helps you to look and feel better in so many ways***.

Water supports your diet and nutrition plan by filling you up, by replacing sugary drinks, and by aiding elimination. It replaces lost fluids after you sleep, then cools and rehydrates you after a workout. In addition, it plays a role in your emotional well-being: sometimes you can feel tired simply because you're mildly dehydrated. A glass of water will do the trick, though, especially after exercise.

~~~~~~~~

Stress is a major factor when it comes to weight gain and other menopausal symptoms, so here are some additional tips to help you *reduce your stress and overcome menopausal fatigue*.

15. **Eat often:** This isn't just a matter of nutrition and metabolism—it is also emotional and psychological. A good way to keep up your energy through the day is to *eat regular meals and healthy snacks every three to four hours*, rather

than a large meal less often. I want to encourage you to **add *energy-sustaining snacks* to your diet,** snacks that provide nutrition as much as they lower stress. These include **whole-grain cereal** with reduced-fat milk or soy; a piece of **whole-grain toast with low/no-sugar peanut butte**r; a piece **of fruit, like a banana**; a **salad with grilled chicken**; a **hard-boiled egg**; a **lean ham and mustard sandwich** on wholegrain bread; a **low-fat yogurt**; and reduced-fat **hummus with celery or sweet pepper**.

16. **Don't overbook:** Stress uses up a lot of energy. ***Embrace relaxation.*** In addition to yoga or Tai Chi, ***add relaxing activities*** throughout your day, like **listening to music, reading,** spending **time with friends,** and receiving **a massage or reflexology** session.

17. **Cut out caffeine***:* The best way to do this is to gradually ***stop having any caffeinated drinks*** (and

that includes coffee, tea, and cola drinks) over a **three-week period**. Try to stay off of caffeine completely for one month, and see if you feel less tired or stressed without it. You may find that stopping caffeine gives you headaches. If this happens, cut down more slowly on the amount of caffeine that you drink.

18. **Drink less alcohol:** Alcohol can **exacerbate the emotional stresses** that accompany menopause. Although a few glasses of wine in the evening may help you to fall asleep, you will sleep less deeply, unfortunately, after drinking alcohol, and you may feel tired the next day, even after a full eight hours of rest. Alcohol can also **promote water retention**, and has been shown to be a **catalyst for mood swings**. Guidelines suggest that women should **not regularly drink more than 2-3 glasses a day.** ("Regularly" means

drinking every day or most days of the week; special occasions are another matter).

19. **Stay connected to your social circle:** Make an effort to *spend time or communicate with people whom you love,* and who love you in return. It will give you a *deep sense of comfort and security* that, in turn, gives you the confidence to tackle menopause.

20. **Cool Off:** There are a few great *strategies that will lower your body temperature* during those years when your hormones are wreaking havoc on your natural thermostat. When you feel less likely to break out in an uncomfortable sweat, you will lower your stress level, too! Working on your weight and adding exercise is going to go a long way towards regulating your hot flashes. **Stop smoking,** if you do: heavy smokers are four times more likely to have hot flashes. Wear **lightweight clothes,** and **dress in layers** of tanks

and cardigans so that you can shed a piece when a hot flash strikes. **Lower your household heat and open a window, plus keep a cool drink** by your side, as hot flashes can be triggered by dehydration. In your journal, also make note of any daily **triggers,** things like spicy foods, caffeine, or alcohol, that you can decrease or eliminate as an experiment in cooler living.

21. **Affirm:** I know I mentioned this in earlier chapters, but it is a tip that I can't underplay. Take those *powerful mini-messages* that move you, and use them to *affirm daily your many reasons for wanting to be healthy and strong*. Affirmations can really help you to stay positive, and to remind you that you definitely have the power to influence your menopausal symptoms. Here are three more of my favorites. Maybe they'll make great additions to your own list!

"Life is either a daring adventure or nothing at all."
—Helen Keller

"You may be faster than me, smarter than me, stronger than me, but you'll never out work me."
—Kris Smith

"It is hard to fail, but it is worse never to have tried to succeed."
—Theodore Roosevelt

# -NINE-

# LET'S GET STARTED!

OK. Now it is time to **begin constructing your very own** Menopause Success Triangle.

Set your goals

And put them into action!

I think that your head is full of ideas and plans, just from reading this book. But I want to offer you two more things.

First, the final chapter of this book is full of some additional resources, links, and information. Please check them out. Then, join our MyMenopauseFix blog and eNewsletter. They will help you to continue to enhance your own "wise menopause" mindset.

Second, I want to offer you a **FREE STRATEGY CALL with a TOP MENOPAUSE COACH.** Sign up online at www.coachwithKris.com, and schedule a session with me or my partner.

Learn about the Coach With Kris process here, too: www.CoachWithKris.com. Read more there about who I am, why you should coach with me, and what you can expect to achieve from this unique and transformational experience.

I share more testimonials on my coaching site as well, plus, once I hear from you, I will schedule a call in order to provide you with more information.

Do you want to enroll in the coaching program?

You'll find a questionnaire/application on that webpage, too, for all prospective clients to submit.

I'm a Certified Master Personal Trainer and Nutritionist, specializing in menopause weight-loss methods. I have also written "The Menopause Cookbook," and "Top 20 Menopause Book List."

Please, go to www.coachwithkris.com to learn more.

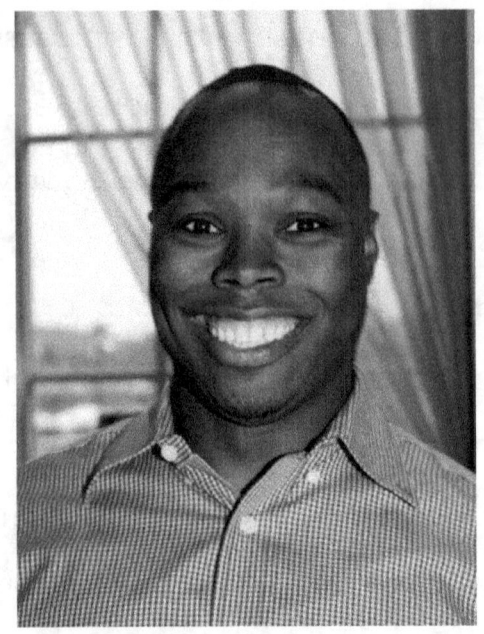

So, let me let you get started today!

**Stay Active.**

**Stay Positive.**

**Embrace your beauty.**

*Kris T. Smith*

## -TEN-

## Recommended Resources and Links

### Kris Smith Additional Resources

"The Menopause Cookbook" by Kris Smith, available at Amazon.com

"Top 20 Menopause Booklist" by Kris Smith, available at www.mymenopausefix.com

### Connect with Kris and the My Menopause Fix Community

**Become a VIP MMF email Subscriber**. Enter your name and email address at http://mymenopausefix.com/. Receive news

and updates that *only VIP members receive*, directly from Kris.

**Facebook Fan Page:** Find us at www.facebook.com/menopausefix. Join the community, and connect with other MMF Members.

**Kris' Menopause Health Podcasts are available on iTunes.** Visit this link: www.mymenopausefix.com/itunes. Kris interviews leading experts in the health and wellness industry regularly.

**Kris' Menopause Health and Training YouTube Channel is also available.** Check out http://www.youtube.com/mymenopausefix. Watch exercise videos, and Kris himself, as he provides inspiration through his unique, positive storytelling.

## Products by Yuri Elkaim, Holistic Nutritionist

www.Yuri Elkaim.org: Yuri Elkaim has helped thousands of people achieve their health goals. He is the leading fitness and nutrition expert in North America, and has innovative views about fitness, as well as many different, popular health programs. His best-known book is *Eating for Energy,* available at Amazon.com. He offers a total wellness cleanse, linked from www.mymenopausefix.com, and full programs with videos and instruction called the "**Yuri Elkaim Fitness Programs for Health Conscious Individuals.**"

"EatingForEnergy"—His 30-Day Raw Food Plan

"Total Wellness Cleanse"—His 30-Day Total Body Cleanse, comprise of all whole foods, and including recipes.

## Clothing

www.attunewomenswear.com: clothing based on TENCEL®, a cutting-edge, naturally-sourced fabric that works to keep you cool. It can be layered to keep you warm, and discretely wicks away even the merest hint of moisture, to keep you comfortable.

www.drybabe.com: Absorbent sleepwear for hot mamas! Uses "absorbing technology" rather than wicking as a better strategy for sleep garments; also can be washed with fabric softener, and won't lose its cooling properties after a hot dryer. Styled for real women—many sizes, fun and flirty.

www.nznature.co.nz: New Zealand Nature offers comfy wicking sleepwear made of *bamboo!* Comfortable, breathable and non-restrictive

## Menopause Resources

www.mymenopausefix.com

www.menopauseatoz.com

www.menopauserus.com

www.34-menopause-symptoms.com

http://360menopause.com

www.menopausegoddessblog.com

## Supplement Sources

BioTrust: www.menopause.biotrust.com

Prograde: www.prograde.com

## Paleo Resources

"ThePaleoCookbook"—Over 390 Recipes

"The21DaySugarDetox"

www.paleodietlifestyle.com

www.thepaleodiet.com

## Oprah's Stress Test

Oprah's online stress test can be found at http://www.oprah.com/spirit/The-Stress-Detector-Test

## ABOUT THE AUTHOR

**Kris T. Smith** is a Certified Master Personal Trainer and Nutritionist specializing in menopause weight-loss methods. Alongside being the author of the *Menopause Cookbook* on Amazon and *The 7-Day Menopause Diet Guide,* Kris and his business partner own a private fitness and nutrition studio in Locust Valley, New *York that services 98% women.*

He has been featured on *WPIX News, News 12 Long Island*, and had many online and offline articles published that share his unique and highly effective weight-loss and nutrition secrets and strategies for women. Since early 1999, Kris has been teaching women around the world how to use simple effective strategies to lose fat, tone and shape their bodies, and feel amazing in their own skin.

Kris has loved being in the gym his entire life, and has always been inspired by entrepreneurs and independent business owners. After developing his skills as a private trainer and fitness manager at the New York Sports Club, he founded his private training facility, and continues to love working with clients and helping others.

After training hundreds and hundreds of women of all ages, he decided to turn his primary professional focus to women over 40, a market for which he had a passion. His goal: to break through the mystery of menopause weight gain. The success "formulas" in this book have been tested on hundreds of women who wanted to increase their metabolism, redesign their bodies, and totally beat the menopause bulge. As they were astounded by their results, he took his Menopause Success Triangle methods to women in multiple states and 3 different countries around the world. He receives raves from everyone who tries his unique fitness, nutrition, and stress-reduction formula.

## Social Media Details: Find Kris Here

**YouTube Channel:**

www.youtube.com/mymenopausefix

**ITunes Podcasts**: www.mymenopausefix.com/itunes

**Facebook Fanpage**:

www.facebook.com/menopausefix

**Twitter**: www.twitter.com/mymenopausefix

**LinkedIn**: Kris T. Smith